Parent Talk

*The Nine Conversations To Have
With Your Aging Loved Ones*

by **G. Scott Middleton**

as an outreach ministry of
Agapé Senior Foundation, Inc.

xulon
ELITE

www.xulonpress.com

The information contained in this book is intended to educate and inform readers, in part by conveying some of the author's experiences through stories and examples. Some names and identifying details have been changed to protect the privacy of individuals. The author has made every effort to ensure that the content of this book was correct at press time, and does not assume and hereby disclaims any liability to any party for any loss, damage or disruption caused by errors or omissions regardless of the cause. This book is not intended to substitute for medical, legal, financial or other professional advice. Persons should always obtain professional consultation specific to their particular needs and issues.

The Cover: The background image is a nine-pointed star. Agapé Senior adopted this symbol as its logo in representation of the nine fruit of the Spirit from the Bible. As excerpted from Galatians 5:22-23:

"But the fruit of the Spirit is love, joy, peace, patience, kindness, goodness, faithfulness, gentleness and self control."

The Author: G. Scott Middleton founded Agapé Senior in February of 1999. Agapé Senior is a network of companies that provide an array of healthcare and related services throughout South Carolina, including assisted living, skilled nursing and rehabilitation, and hospice. Additional provisions include services such as physician care, pharmacy and medical equipment. As a believer in comprehensive solutions, Scott also incorporated independent living, insurance and real estate services into the network to assist seniors during their transition.

Agapé Senior holds itself as a faith-based organization. The network now cares for more than 1,200 residents and hospice patients, provides services to hundreds of other customers, and employs more than 1,000 dedicated team members.

Scott holds a Bachelor of Science in financial accounting from Winthrop University, a Master of Health Administration from the University of South Carolina, and a Master of Divinity from Emory University. Reverend Middleton is an ordained United Methodist minister. He is also a board member of the South Carolina State Chamber of Commerce.

Dedication

I would like to dedicate this book to all who are, or have been, a part of the Agapé Family; from residents and their family members to staff and partners, for it is their stories that inspired *The Nine Conversations*. I would especially like to thank my parents, David and Denise Middleton, my in-laws Frank and Jess Cook, and my grandmother Martha Middleton who, through their progressions in life, have taught me so much about being a responsible adult child of aging loved ones. And most of all, I must thank my dear wife, Evelyn, and my children, Greg and Sara, who have provided unyielding support throughout my education, my career changes, and all the opportunities that life has afforded me to further our ministry to senior adults.

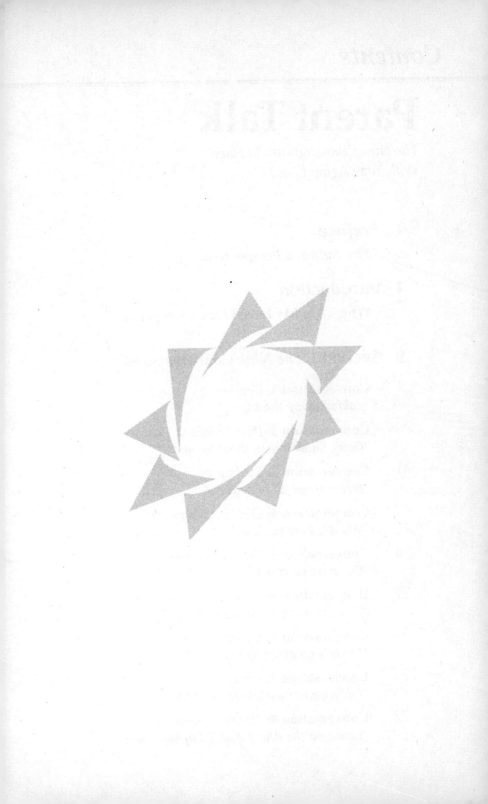

Contents

Parent Talk

*The Nine Conversations To Have
With Your Aging Loved Ones*

The Author's Perspective...

I am grateful that you have chosen to read this book. My purpose in sharing this information is to enlighten you regarding some of the more difficult decisions related to caring for senior adults and to assist you in preparing to address these challenges. After the Introduction, I have divided the body of the book into four main sections. In addition to *The Nine Conversations* in Section I, I have included three supplemental sections – Residential and Care Options, Health Issues, and Financial Planning. I have also provided a reference section that consists of citations, a glossary, and a listing of helpful contact information for various agencies and organizations.

Before we delve into the subject of caring for seniors, I would like to share some information concerning my background, my perspective on life and why I felt compelled to write this book.

I know I am imperfect, yet I constantly seek purity in my life, as I strive to be a better man of God. I am extremely busy, yet ever mindful of those dearest to me, as I am a committed son, husband and father. I struggle with dyslexia, yet I am a passionate reader who makes his way through some 50 books, numerous periodicals and web publications each year, as I aspire to learn all that I possibly can. I have Attention Deficit Disorder, yet harness enough focus to immerse myself in accounting records and spreadsheet budgets for hours, as I am a person of numbers.

I have always loved numbers. When I was a child, my teacher asked the class to count as high as we could by writing numbers. Most of the students made it to 100, while I counted into the thousands. I could not stop!

Numbers continue to fascinate me, especially when I see how they are used in every aspect of life. Take the number "nine". Not only does it possess many unique mathematical characteristics, it is also commonly referenced in our American culture: "cloud nine," "love potion number nine," "dressed to the nines," "the bottom of the ninth," "the whole nine yards," etc.

My company, Agapé Senior, adopted the nine-pointed star as its logo. However, the significance of "nine" in this application lies in its representation of the fruit of the Spirit from the fifth chapter of Galatians. Verses 22 and 23 tell us, "The fruit of the Spirit is love, joy, peace, patience, kindness, goodness, faithfulness, gentleness and self control." The fruit of the Spirit symbolizes the virtues we embrace at Agapé; and we, as an organization, hold these values as our guide in the daily care of our residents and patients.

Several years before I felt called into senior healthcare, I attended Emory University's Candler School of Theology. Subsequently, I served as a Methodist minister in the rural Lowcountry of South Carolina. It was there that my life was literally changed as I witnessed the plight of an elderly couple in my parish.

He was a tall and rugged farmer who had worked the land his entire life and always managed for himself and his family. He had developed what is now commonly known as Alzheimer's disease. She was a feeble yet devoted wife, determined to do her best in seeking care for her beloved husband. She entrusted her loved one to South Carolina's mental hospital, as was common in those days, and was assured he would be much better when she returned to visit him. After a few restless weeks, she made her return journey to the hospital in Columbia. As she anxiously made the turn from the corridor into his room, her glowing excitement quickly darkened. To her heart-broken sorrow, he lay strapped to his bed, medicated to the point that he was almost non-responsive. Without speaking a word, she unbuckled the straps, helped her husband to a wheelchair, and took him home. At that moment, she assumed the full burden of caring for her husband on her own for the rest of his life. Despite his episodes of confusion and violent outbursts, to the point that she sometimes had to lock herself into a bedroom to protect her own well-being, she never wavered and cared for him until his death.

During my 10 years as a minister, several troubling experiences, such as seeing that precious woman's struggles, made me realize *there must be a better way.* This is when I felt God's calling into a ministry of caring for senior adults.

As I continued to explore this calling through extensive prayer and soul searching, I enrolled in The University of South Carolina's Master of Health Administration program. Over the next few years, I gained invaluable knowledge regarding the workings of the healthcare industry. The more I observed, the more I discovered how to overcome many firmly entrenched obstacles to providing better care.

When I founded Agapé Senior in February of 1999, I had a vision of building that *better way.* This vision has since been continuously reshaped by innumerable insights gained through interactions with residents, patients, peers and experts throughout the senior care industry. And while I have been blessed with many successes, I have also learned that this *better way* will forever be a work in progress, because people, along with their needs, are constantly changing in response to the world around us. Which brings us to now, when God's calling and my experiences working with senior adults since that time have inspired me to share my realizations through the writing of this book.

Why I Am My Loved One's Keeper...

From the moment we are born, we seek a higher degree of independence. In fact, the process of birth itself is an assertion of independence as it signifies that the newborn no longer depends on the mother's body. From our first steps, to our first day of school, the first time we drive a car, go off to college, get married or receive that first big promotion, we are in a continuous progression toward independence. To succeed on our own merits and to live by our own means is the basis of a capitalistic society. Most of us feel the need to prove to the world around us that we can stand on our own.

No matter what our age, it seems we all desire independence. Yet, at the same time, we deliberately seek to establish relationships that, ironically, create dependence within our lives. As these relationships evolve, they give us strength, comfort, insight and eventually interdependence. They present to us opportunities for personal growth. As a pastor, I have been questioned on a handful of occasions as to the true importance of the church. Some have said, "I feel so much closer to God when I am outside amidst God's creations, on the lake fishing or hiking through the woods. I feel His presence more so when I am alone and quiet. So, why do I need to go to church?" My answer is simple. The presence of God is certainly made known in the serenity of one's reverent solitude; however, God is nonetheless present in a powerful and strengthening way that is revealed only when we gather together with others to worship. Remember the assurance we are given through Christ in Matthew 18:20, "For where two or three are gathered in my name, there am I among them." God recognizes the value of certain dependencies and instills in each of us a sense of need for others in our lives. In the end, we can achieve the highest *practical* level of independence only by understanding and embracing our dependence on those around us to enhance every aspect of our lives.

The truth is our quality of life can suffer dramatically if we deprive ourselves of adequate socialization. But in the case of a declining senior adult, especially when the spouse is no longer living, the lack of interaction with others poses one of the greatest and most debilitating threats to their well-being — *isolation*. The lack of adequate socialization is the silent enemy of an aging senior that too many "caretakers" fail to understand or consider. Here lies one of the biggest drawbacks to home health care. It tends to discourage "getting out of the house" and does little to counteract the loss of socialization. Isolation has a significant adverse effect on a person's psychological health and can quickly bring on depression and all the physical issues that compound this sad and often preventable condition. Unfortunately, failure to manage decline in an effective and timely manner often results in isolation, thus the loss of independence is accelerated. As portrayed by Tom Hanks' character in the movie Cast Away, living in complete isolation can, over time, threaten one's sanity. If we remain isolated for too long, we will lose our desire to interact and eventually our ability to thrive.

One concern regarding healthcare reform legislation is that it subsidizes home services for seniors rather than funds assisted living and skilled nursing homes, thereby supporting decisions that contribute to isolation. While I am in favor of individual choice and realize that a significant number of seniors would choose to remain at home, the reality is that many cannot safely do so. If ailing seniors are going to be encouraged to stay at home via the subsidization of in-home care, then there should be competent oversight for their well-being.

There is no doubt that the considerations of caring for seniors are complex and challenging, and can occupy a great deal of time. And that is a resource that no one seems to have enough of these days. Many of us are part of what is known as the *Sandwich Generation*. We are supporting children while also becoming caretakers for our aging parents. A recent AARP study estimates that 44 percent of Americans between the ages of 45 and 55 are caring for aging loved ones as well as for children under the age of 21.[1] While our teenagers are seeking to establish their own independence, our parents are becoming increasingly dependent on us for many of their needs. In many ways, our roles as parents are the polar opposite of our roles as children. Yet, they can be uncannily similar. As our children continue to grow and learn, our parents, even though they may remain active and alert, are experiencing some of the early signs of decline. While both children and parents long for independence, children strive to *acquire* it, while parents struggle to *retain* it. There are times when each of us, as both a parent and a child, must intervene in order to ensure the safety and well-being of our children and our parents. Despite the realities of decline, most parents tend to hold fast to the opinion that, because they have cared for themselves all of their lives, they do not need anyone to tell them what to do. Or do they?

One of the greatest challenges of raising children is learning to differentiate between the times when we should actively parent and the times when we need to let go and give them room to grow on their own. Similarly, when we are facing the task of caring for aging parents, there comes a time when we must be comfortable *parenting our parents*. We need to ensure their safety and well-being, while still considering their quality of life. In other words, we may have to *limit* their freedoms in order to *preserve* their freedom. We, as their children and caretakers, have to learn to recognize when we need to intervene.

When a senior's independence or freedom is first compromised, friends and neighbors often help compensate by providing transportation and diversion. But in almost all cases, these efforts weigh heavy on the well-intentioned caregivers, and the full burden suddenly transfers to family members. Many of them find themselves ill-prepared to deal with the difficult questions and challenges that arise, often in rapid succession.

A time-honored lesson involving the caretaking of a senior can be found in the Biblical story of Ruth and her mother-in-law, Naomi. In studying God's word, I find no more fitting example of love, appreciation and respect for older adults than in the story of these two women. Following her husband's death, Ruth easily could have returned to her native land to be cared for by her own family, but opted instead for a very meager lifestyle that allowed her to look after Naomi. Because of Ruth's loyalty, God showed favor on her and led her to Boaz, a well-to-do man from Bethlehem. Having been deeply moved by Ruth's devotion to care for her mother-in-law, Boaz was impassioned to know this woman of such great character. This led to the eventual marriage of Ruth and Boaz and, subsequently, to Naomi's being cared for in the finest manner.

Taking care of an elderly loved one does not mean you have to take a vow of poverty or completely give up your life in order to be a full-time caregiver. In fact, it shouldn't if you learn *what to expect* and *how to plan wisely.* In the story of Ruth, Naomi insisted that Ruth return to her own family, for she knew there awaited a full and rich life for Ruth. But Ruth, in knowing what was truly best for Naomi, remained with her. It was this selfless decision made on behalf of her loved one that eventually yielded bountiful blessings for both Ruth and Naomi.

In much the same sense, moving a loved one into a retirement community, assisted living or nursing facility can, in fact, be one of the most caring actions we can take on their behalf. Protecting a parent from engaging in potentially harmful activities is a gesture of love. Although these and other necessary interventions may not be popular or easy, they are responsible and loving.

A person with aging parents typically procrastinates on major decisions about the long term care of their parents. Quite often this is due to some degree of denial which adds to the difficulty of making timely and objective choices regarding our parents' lives. Avoiding the important issues we need to consider or even refusing to engage in the thought process is an easy mistake to make. It's a lot like having the conversations with children about sex or drugs. While these are in many ways challenging topics to discuss, the sooner we can speak candidly about these subjects, the more effective it will be and the more comfortable it will become. Having ongoing conversations is a critical part of this process because there is so much information that needs to be considered. Don't leave it to chance; don't wait until that moment of urgency when everything seems confusing and chaotic. Don't allow your inhibitions to put you in a predicament you may regret for the rest of your life. Be fair to your parents. Talk to them while they are physically, mentally and emotionally able to be a constructive part of planning their long term care. Educate yourself now! Help your parents understand all the options and likelihoods. Don't let them speak in terms of *absolutes* about what they will or will not do. And don't make promises you know are not in their best interest. Be compassionate out of respect, but be forthright out of necessity. And don't lose sight of your ultimate goal — *to help them live better!*

God has put each of us on this earth with many purposes, one of which is to care for our parents as they age and decline. What the scripture is telling us through Ruth's story is that we should know and appreciate the blessings and wisdom of those who have lived many years before us. Every human being is created in the image of God and deserves to be loved and cared for during the latter years of their life. We should constantly hold each of them in a position of respect and dignity and care for their physical, emotional and spiritual needs. While our good deeds and loyalty may not yield us earthly riches, they will, when rendered with a pure heart, place us in the midst of God's blessings.

Section I

The Nine Conversations

Then and Now...

As you read this book, I hope that you will be able to dispel any misconceptions you may hold about long term care and to gain a clear understanding of what you need to know in order to make sound decisions on behalf of your loved one.

One of the most curious aspects of history is how certain theories and beliefs were held to be *absolute* for so long. Yet when we look back on the past, the fallacies inherent in those theories and beliefs seem so obvious. It sometimes makes you wonder, "How could we not have realized that?" For instance, from the days before Jesus walked the earth and for many centuries after his death, the greatest scientific minds on earth thought the world was flat.

In 1847, a Hungarian physician discovered that the death rate in his hospital dropped significantly after doctors were required to wash their hands following autopsies. [2] Elsewhere, however, doctors ignored these findings, ridiculing the notion that illness could be prevented simply by washing hands.

Until the 1950s, cigarette smoking was not only considered acceptable from the standpoint of health, but was actually *prescribed* by physicians to "calm the nerves." Even after it was scientifically proven that smoking posed numerous health risks, there were some physicians who continued to endorse smoking as a "safe practice."

When I was a child growing up in the 1960s, I went on several long trips with my family. My brother and I would ride in the back of the station wagon. We would jump back and forth from the back seat to the cargo area, set up board games and play all over the car. Today, I would be arrested if I allowed my children to ride unrestrained. It was not that my mother and father were bad parents; it was just that the importance of seat belts was not promoted as widely as it is today. Yet in the late 1950s, crash tests clearly showed that seat belts saved lives. Even though the information was known and available, we as a society did not make the issue a priority until years later. Nonetheless, from 1975 to 2006, seat belts saved the lives of more than 200,000 people in the United States alone. [3]

Throughout history, medical research has been marked by the establishment and, often times, subsequent rejection of diagnoses and treatments. An accepted medical practice for centuries involved the use of leeches in treating patients who were diagnosed with the condition of "excess blood." For many decades, prevailing Western medical procedures involved the administration of antibiotics at the onset of any and every illness; but we now know that our bodies can become immune to antibiotics if they are used too often. More recently, millions of people died from what was initially described as a "strain of killer pneumonia." In the 1980s scientists discovered that the true cause of the mysterious sicknesses and deaths, the HIV virus, was transmitted through bodily fluids.

The list goes on. The point is that throughout history, our beliefs and knowledge have evolved through a series of revelations. The same holds true for the evolution of senior adult care. Continued discoveries and evolutions have greatly improved the knowledge base and practice standards in long term care. For example, in the 1970s health professionals, would physically restrain older adults who were at risk of falling as a matter of protection; we now realize that restraints limit the use of muscles to the point that the body weakens further, and the lack of movement can lead to bed sores and other skin and tissue damage.

Regardless of how far the long term care industry has evolved, I still hear too many people make comments like, "Don't put me in one of those depressing old nursing homes," or "You'll never get me into one of those places." While this may have been understandable in the past, today it is both troubling and misguided. It's troubling because it tells me that too few people are learning about long term care options for their parents. It's misguided because there are now a variety of great care options available. Admittedly, there was a time when the old, institutionalized nursing homes of the past were "the norm." Even today, facilities exist that fit the dated nursing home stereotype. But it is sad that this outdated perception characterizes the industry in the minds of many people who *still* don't understand how much the industry has changed. If we refuse to educate ourselves regarding available options for our parents, then their needs may not be fully met. In so doing, we will very likely have denied them readily available quality care.

When I think back on the experiences that led me to this line of work, I am amazed at the changes that have come to the senior-care industry over the past 25 years.

In the early 1980s, while serving as a minister, I led visitation at a nursing home not far from our church. I recall the cold cinder block building, the long poorly lit hallways and the molding ceiling tiles. No matter where I walked in the facility, I could not get away from the overpowering odors. The atmosphere was depressing. The image that is foremost in my memory is one of the facility's residents lined up and down the hallway, stretching out their arms to us as we walked by. Some cried out for help. I could not begin to understand what was occurring. My surroundings literally scared me. I later learned that the residents were lined up as a convenience for the facility's doctor, so that "check-ups" would not be so time-consuming. In disbelief, I thought to myself, "What about consideration and respect for the residents? It is a 'convenience' for the doctor?"

This was one of a handful of experiences that led me into senior healthcare, and to knowing, *"There must be a better way."*

Today, there *is!* When I founded Agapé Senior in 1999, I set out to create that *better way.* My dream was to build a network of long term care services that would transcend those institutional buildings and dated practices. I envisioned beautifully decorated, lively facilities with care services that render compassion and dignity. I wanted to create an environment that holds God as our enabler and ultimate caregiver.

I also envisioned care options that meet seniors where they are in their progression and strategies that encourage our residents to interact with others. I wanted to help residents maintain their independence and dignity. That's why it is important to offer so many different types of care, from independent living to assisted living and nursing facilities, and differing levels of services and amenities within each of these options.

A New Beginning

From firsthand knowledge I understand how different today's senior care options are from those of the past. A burning desire to bring about positive changes for this industry is, in essence, what brought me into this line of work. For anyone who still mistakenly thinks that long term care marks the end of life, I would like to introduce you to a dear lady who touched our lives and made her assisted living experience the *start* of a life of new opportunities.

———————————————

After retiring in Texas and then living with a daughter in North Carolina, Mildred Memler and her husband, John, came to Agapé's original campus in West Columbia, South Carolina. Soon after her arrival in 1997, it became obvious that Mildred was a woman with a wide range of interests and an irrepressible spirit. She was a former school teacher, 4-H leader and Sunday School teacher, as well as a poet, writer and painter.

At the age of 89, she quickly made a name for herself when she set up a small art studio in the corner of her living room and began creating an inspiring array of oil paintings. Interest in her artwork quickly grew, and soon Mildred was selling her paintings to other residents, staff members, and people in the community.

Mildred was an active participant in Agapé Senior's daily exercise program. She was approached by her peers and asked to help direct the classes. Mildred accepted the challenge and went on to lead a variety of exercise sessions, including tai chi, for more than a decade.

In 2001, John, Mildred's loving husband for 69 years, died from complications related to Parkinson's disease. One surviving daughter, six grandchildren, and eleven great grandchildren shared in the loss. A time of mourning followed; however, Mildred soon rediscovered her vigor and plunged anew into her many duties and regimens.

Before coming to Agapé, Mildred and her husband endured the loss of a daughter to bone cancer. The daughter had begun a family genealogy project years before, but the work remained unfinished at her death. She left behind folders full of hand-written notes, which had been boxed up and tucked away. Mildred sent for the boxes, determined to see her daughter's dream come to fruition. With the help of a "tech-savvy" grandson, she learned to use a personal computer. Focusing her considerable energies on a labor of love, she meticulously typed all of her daughter's notes into the computer. She then summoned the grandson once again so that she could learn about the Internet and further research the family history.

In the summer of 2000, Mildred proudly displayed the final product of the mother-daughter journey, a printed version of the family tree, which covered an entire wall of her apartment.

Armed with computer skills and a desire to contribute, Mildred next volunteered to create and distribute facility newsletters, phone lists and newcomers' guides. Mildred also began to create and print informational flyers and signs. She was soon put in charge of the facility's bulletin boards. Within a remarkably short time, Mildred had become a repository of information on Agapé. Always willing to share her knowledge of and appreciation for the facility and its diverse population of residents, Mildred served as Agapé Senior's first hospitality committee leader—to the surprise of no one.

After her momentous 100th birthday, Mildred sat down with an administrator from Agapé and reflected on her nineties and what those years might have been like if she had chosen to remain at home, "The stress and difficulty of being home alone would have been overwhelming. I have lived this long because of not having to deal with that extra stress. I'm very happy living at Agapé." When *asked to name memorable events that took place during her years at Agapé, Mildred answered, "The growth at West Columbia and with all of Agapé." Mildred also remarked on an important constant during her years at Agapé — her fellowship with other residents. "We are all a family at Agapé and we all look after each other."*

During her 13 rewarding and enriching years in South Carolina, Mildred lived in four different Agapé Senior facilities and took advantage of Agapé Senior's skilled nursing, rehabilitative, palliative and hospice services.

In January of 2010, Mildred Memler quietly passed away under the care of Agapé's hospice. Her 101 years left a legacy of life lived to the fullest.

Mrs. Memler's story is one of inspiration and revelation to everyone. Her life at Agapé is a shining example of how a nurturing environment can enable seniors to flourish, not merely survive.

As seniors age and their abilities decline, they have to become more selective in what they do, or else they run an increased risk of incident or injury. When these progressions begin, decisions can be made more effectively and objectively if your parent is already comfortable openly discussing these matters. Following are *the nine conversations* that each of us should have with our aging loved ones. Each of these conversations includes a story related to senior care challenges. Although the names in the remaining stories have been changed, the accounts are based on actual events. These first nine chapters will introduce the issues that should be discussed with your parents and will help you address these subjects in a candid, yet loving manner.

"Taking away the keys..."

*O*ne of my employees, Betty, has a father who is 85 years old. He lives at home and is fairly independent. Although he walks with a cane, he still works on the family farm.

His family is very attentive. Over the years they have prided themselves on "taking care of Dad." Betty would usually swing by the house and bring her father a hot lunch. She and her brother juggled the doctors' appointments. Her brother gave him a paycheck for helping out on the farm and the family tried very hard to help dad keep his independence. However, by looking at Dad through "rose-colored glasses", the family almost cost him his life. They never had any conversations with Dad about his aging issues or his limitations because they were "afraid to go there." Betty's father still drove to town once or twice a week to get groceries or a hair-cut. One day that all changed...

Betty had driven to the house one day to deliver lunch. Her father was not home. She called her brother to see if he knew where their Dad was. Her brother wasn't sure — "Maybe he went to town."

After waiting a few minutes, Betty left the lunch on the kitchen table with a note; she had to get back to work. She hopped in her car and started toward the office. It was a calm and sunny day.

After driving a short distance, Betty noticed a truck heading her way. When she saw that the truck had crossed the center line and was coming right at her, she blew the horn and frantically swerved out of the truck's path. She thought to herself, "What's wrong with him?"

To her horror, she realized that the driver was... HER DAD! Betty had to pull over because she had a knot in her stomach. Her father just kept driving and never realized that he had almost killed his own daughter.

Questions rushed through her mind: What if it had been someone else that he met in the road? What if he had killed somebody? What if he had been killed? How long has he been driving like this?

The events of that day convinced the entire family that Dad could no longer be allowed to drive. It was a tough decision, but it would have been considerably easier if the family had talked about it first and had given their father time to prepare. The sudden change in his lifestyle made the transition difficult for him to accept.

The time will come, if it hasn't already, when establishing some road rules for Mom or Dad will be the most important health and safety decision you face. Think about it. A car accident can kill quicker than any disease.

This will, no doubt, be one of the more challenging conversations because driving a vehicle has such a direct impact on independence. As long as your parent can drive, they can pretty much come and go as they please; that is empowering. The pertinent question to pose here is, "Can they still drive safely?" The trouble is that the answer isn't always simple or clear. It's no secret that as we age, our sense of awareness loses its sharpness and our reflexes are not as quick as they once were. However, much of the challenge lies in the fact that some of these issues progress slowly, making them more difficult to detect, thus making them easier for the parent to deny. Many seniors mistakenly think that if they just slow it down when behind the wheel, things will be O.K. This line of thinking is misguided — a slower driver is not necessarily a safer, or even better, driver. In fact, driving 45 miles per hour on the interstate is more likely to cause frustration among other drivers and result in their taking more and unnecessary risks while trying to maneuver around the slow, impeding vehicle.

The best way to avoid an accident while operating a vehicle is to be an alert, defensive driver. Defense relies on the ability to observe and predict what is going on around you (i.e. awareness) and being able to react quickly (i.e. reflexes) to other drivers' carelessness or negligence. In many cases, these are capabilities that too many senior drivers no longer possess. Split seconds can mean the difference between life and death when struggling to control a 3,000-pound vehicle.

We need to keep a close watch on the progression of our parents' physical limitations. We also must have enough foresight to be mindful of how the eventual loss of this important freedom will affect their lives and feelings of self worth. The most effective approach in addressing this matter is to begin the transition process early so that it can take place over a period of time. The threat to an aging adult's perspective of independence can be made less of an issue if changes in their routines take place gradually. So, how do you change their routines? You invest a little time and apply some good old-fashioned strategy.

As our parents age, it is a good idea to start limiting not only the places *where* they drive, but also the times *when* they drive. Avoiding morning and evening rush hour is a logical starting point. Restricting driving at night, on interstate highways and transporting passengers could be a second phase. Many of the proven strategies used with teenage drivers also make sense with seniors.

Any activity that allows you to observe their driving abilities or that decreases their driving time can be beneficial. Perhaps you could meet your parent at their house and ride with them to church or to the doctor's office. Watch for indications of how alert they are while driving. Are they focused? Do they react quickly enough to changing conditions or situations? Also, do they remember the directions to these routine locations? A subtle strategy for decreasing your parent's driving time is to coordinate your schedule so that you can drive your parent to their favorite destinations. "Hey Mom, I'm going shopping Saturday. Why don't you go with me and we can stop for breakfast on the way." Store and mall parking lots are among the most dangerous and confusing places to operate a vehicle, so this strategy can have significant benefits.

As the parent's routines change, an important transition begins to evolve. As driving becomes less a part of their routine, they may not feel as much of a need or desire to drive. Once this starts to take place, they will be more receptive to discussing times of day, and traffic and weather conditions in which they probably shouldn't drive, and hopefully even agree to setting some guidelines.

There are, of course, some situations that do not allow for a progressive approach and require quicker and more direct interventions. The period immediately following a major illness is a time when you should monitor their recovery very closely as it relates to whether or not they are able to continue driving. Regardless, this is usually a good time to go ahead and discuss the probable need to limit driving from that point forward.

Because an aging parent is often most resistant to advice or declarations coming from their child, don't discount the potential effectiveness of utilizing *the system*. Doctors are trained to recognize conditions that could make it unsafe for your parent to engage in activities such as driving. They can then write a letter to that effect to the local Department of Motor Vehicles. Many states' DMV's will then require that your parent's driving skills be re-examined. By taking this approach, the "trained professional" breaks the ice, allowing you to be a source of consoling reinforcement. In South Carolina, re-examination may be recommended by a medical professional, family member or a law enforcement official.

The main purpose of this section is to encourage you to be aware of your parent's driving capabilities and activities. Not too long ago, I spoke with a family about their mother who had recently moved into one of our facilities. As they were cleaning out their mom's home, they discovered several traffic citations stuffed back in one of her drawers.

The lesson here is not to make any assumptions and never to take anything for granted when it comes to a parent's driving habits. Did they pass their last eye exam? Is their driver's license still current and valid? Many states require older drivers to renew their licenses more frequently than others. In South Carolina, persons age 65 and older must renew their driver's license every five years, as opposed to every ten years for younger drivers. If the answer to these types of questions is "No," then it's probably time to *take away the keys*. Once you do, don't leave anything to chance. Take the extra step to disable the vehicle, because a determined parent will definitely remember where they hid the extra key. If you don't take charge when the signs are there, you are, in essence, giving your parent a "license to kill."

Driving Exercise

Observe your parent while they:

- Drive from home to the doctor's office, pharmacy, grocery store and church.

- Practice parking in at least two of these places.

- Negotiate intersections with traffic signals.

- Make left-hand turns.

Do your best to set them up for success, not failure. Schedule the exercise for times with lighter traffic. Set the route so that they encounter various conditions, and see how the changes affect their driving skills.

"Don't know much about *'ology'*..."

*A*n old friend of mine, Danny, recently called to relay a story about his elderly father. His father, Roger, had suffered two heart attacks and an aneurism in recent years. He also suffered from high blood pressure. But unfortunately Roger had not been truthful with Danny.

Roger had been hospitalized three times in fairly rapid succession, but was now living at home by himself. Over the past two years, Danny had faithfully checked on his father—by phone and in person. Danny traveled frequently for work, but was convinced that he was "on top of things" regarding his father's health. Whenever Danny asked his father about check-ups, medications and doctors' instructions, Roger was quick to reply with reassurances and specifics. Roger's replies were thorough and convincing. The problem was, Roger was lying through his teeth.

As a child of the Great Depression, Roger had learned early in life that money and possessions were not to be squandered. The formal education of Roger and his siblings concluded after elementary school. Full-time work on the family farm awaited them after the sixth grade. Throughout his long life, Roger kept the memories of that meager existence close and never surrendered a nickel without a struggle.

After his hospitalizations, Roger had shown up for initial follow-up visits with the doctor and followed all *instructions regarding medication and therapy. However, after these initial follow-up visits, Roger cancelled all other appointments and stopped getting his prescriptions refilled even though money and insurance were available to cover the majority of expenses without Danny's assistance. The issue at hand was what Roger considered frivolous spending. Roger did not see the necessity or value of continuing the medical care that had been prescribed for him.*

The inevitable phone call came as Danny was preparing for a business trip to Denver. One of Roger's friends called from the hospital to inform Danny that his father had been admitted and was in "rough shape." As Danny frantically drove to the hospital, he began calling doctors' offices in an attempt to get "up to speed" on his dad's condition. After two phone calls, a slow and painful realization hit Danny. Roger had not been to see a doctor of any kind in more than two years.

Danny made it to the hospital in time to say his goodbyes, but his father soon lost consciousness and died two days later.

Many senior adults have multiple doctors and usually end up seeing only specialists (i.e. cardiologist, urologist, etc.). Mistakenly, they no longer feel a need to see a family doctor. As your parents start to decline, and especially when they are seeing specialists, it is extremely important that the family physician be involved in the management of health issues. One of the biggest problems in managing a senior's health issues is that while each of the specialists is probably prescribing at least one medication, all too often no one is monitoring *the big picture*. Effectively caring for a declining senior can be a complex undertaking, due to the presence of numerous chronic issues. This is complicated even further by the potential for damaging drug interactions that exist when multiple doctors are individually prescribing numerous medicines. Geriatric physicians are specifically trained in dealing with seniors and the existence of numerous chronic health issues. Unfortunately, certified geriatricians are few and far between. There are, however, a number of informed internists, family physicians, nurse practitioners and physician assistants who have the training and experience necessary to care for seniors with multiple diagnoses. The key is to be sure the practitioner who is treating your parent possesses the right skills, knowledge and willingness to manage all the details of treatment.

On the other hand, there are too many seniors who avoid visits to a doctor all together because they don't think there is anything that the doctor can do, or they simply may not want to know the status of their health. When seniors are in tune with their own bodies, they have the necessary knowledge that enables them to be an active part of formulating their own health plan; it helps keep them in control. By engaging in conversations with medical professionals, they can come to understand the value of exercise and what exercise can do to enhance their ability to enjoy life. For example, bone deterioration is a common and debilitating issue for many seniors. Exercise that strengthens muscles can help enable the senior to remain active longer. They can also choose to seek therapies that enable them to function better and lessen the likelihood or severity of falls. Medicare "Part B" will pay for outpatient and home health therapy several times a year if ordered by the doctor. This constant attention to physical exercise could add many productive years to your parent's life. Find creative ways to help your parent associate a better quality of life with seeing a physician on a regular basis. *Awareness* should be an asset, not a burden.

The frequency of visits should increase with the number and severity of health issues. Some physicians follow a particular guideline: for every decade a person has lived, there is likely a health issue that needs to be identified, monitored and treated. It is very common for seniors to have health issues and start gradually slowing down well before they realize they are sick.

By the time they realize they are ill, it can often be too late for effective treatment. Early warning signs of oncoming or potential health problems are often discovered during routine doctor's visits. Regular visits will also allow you and your parent to stay abreast of their conditions and understand what is going on inside their body.

Once you are able to get your parent to see a physician on a regular basis, you will then need to guide them to understand *how* and *why* certain decisions will need to be made regarding care and treatment. What should they expect over the coming years, and what do they want?

Physicians *practice* medicine. They do so because no one doctor possesses complete expertise in all areas. Each person's body has a unique biological makeup, giving it its own set of characteristics and conditions. As a result, medicines work differently in different people. Medications are most effective if an individual's response is monitored frequently and dosages are adjusted accordingly, rather than being prescribed by some *typical standard*. Sometimes, a low dose of medicine will actually be more effective, and is preferable to higher doses. People respond to treatments and therapies differently. Therefore, practitioners should constantly seek to find the right solution for each patient. Providing the most effective care, especially when managing numerous chronic issues, is always a work in progress.

In addition to obtaining practical experience, a good practitioner is constantly seeking to gain more knowledge. Most people choose a family doctor because of the location, convenience and personality of the physician; some make their choice based on the physician's reputation in the community. I pick doctors based largely on what they are *willing to learn*, not just what they know. Practitioners should continuously read, study the results of the latest research, and collaborate with other health professionals. A willingness to learn, combined with experience in caring for patients with similar health issues leads to familiarity expertise and a greater level of proficiency

What are the important considerations when choosing a physician? Do they work with a lot of older patients? Sometimes, a question as simple as, "How many of your patients are over the age of 65?" can provide some insight as to the practitioner's familiarity with treating senior adults, and at least open the door to more discussion. Do they have experience working in a nursing facility or hospital? Other questions include, "Will they communicate frequently with your parent's specialists?" and "Will they listen before they prescribe?" If the answers to these kinds of questions are "Yes" then they will likely have been exposed to many older adults and therefore be more familiar with the complications involved in treating multiple diagnoses.

When consulting with a new physician, realize that their days are very busy and often chaotic. It is prudent to take advantage of every available opportunity to grab their attention and have them focus on your parent's conditions. Be sure to get your parent's medical history to the physician a few days in advance of the initial appointment. Hopefully this will give them time to have read over this information and become familiar with your parent's conditions. The more detailed your parent's medical history, the better equipped the physician will be to move toward the most effective plan of care. Identify the best person in the office to facilitate communication.

When you arrive for your parent's appointment, don't go in empty-handed. Carry a copy of the medical history with you and place it in the hand of the physician yourself. If they state that they already had a chance to review the copy you sent earlier, then you have a good feel for where things are in terms of the physician's knowledge of your parent. If not, you may want to open your discussion with reference to the medical history to establish a baseline. An effective way to introduce your parent's health issues is to hand your physician a list of pertinent questions concerning your parent's health. It is important to spend time talking about health issues in general, touch on specific concerns, and also address your parent's wishes regarding life support and end of life care. Even persons in excellent health should make this type of information known to their physician and family.

I would advise anyone who is assisting or caring for senior parents to put together an envelope for each parent that contains all of their pertinent medical information. This Lifeline Information for Emergencies Packet (LIFE Packet) should contain information such as personal data (name, address, birth date, social security number, etc.), list of medical conditions, medications, health insurance information, living will, power of attorney designation, emergency contacts, etc. The packet should read "EMERGENCY INFO" in large bold letters and bear the owner's name. Be sure that the LIFE Packet is kept in a secure location that is known to several immediate family members. The contents of your parent's LIFE Packet should include most, if not all, of the same pertinent information as is needed for initial visits with any medical service provider.

The reality of effective senior medical care is that, as a person ages and declines, a gradual transition needs to take place if they want to get the most out of their lives. By no means does this suggest they should give up. It simply means that they, and we (if we *truly* wish to help them), should understand that the likelihood of achieving certain health outcomes will continue to change; therefore their expectations, choices and goals will need to change as a result.

Again, accepting this progression is *not* a sign of giving up. In fact, it's a conscious and proactive strategy to help them get all they can out of life. We should always consider their quality of life within any decision regarding medical care. When an infection or viral condition arises, we should aggressively treat the issue with the goal of completely eliminating the problem as promptly as possible. There are times when more aggressive treatments such as surgery are preferable. However, we should consider these more aggressive options in relation to how they will affect the overall *quality* in their lives.

Most physicians and insurance companies will want to exhaust medicinal treatment options before considering surgeries or other remedies. While this is fairly common in the practice of medicine, there are situations when this approach is probably not the most prudent.

It is important to remember many older adults generally have multiple health issues, requiring multiple medications. As a result, the potential exists for side effects or interactions that might exacerbate health problems. One specific example would be that medications for urinary incontinence often cause dizziness. Seniors who suffer from urinary tract infections will often find themselves rushing to the restroom because their bladders are overactive. When this haste is coupled with dizziness, the potential for injury is increased exponentially. For seniors with chronic urinary difficulties, electrical stimulation therapy or implant surgery could strengthen the bladder and could very well eliminate the need for medication. Sometimes a more aggressive, non-medicinal plan can affect improved environmental safety *and* quality of life. Learn all you can about your parent's conditions and don't be afraid to discuss your findings with the physician.

The key in this example is that the benefits to your parent in terms of safety and comfort could greatly outweigh the inconvenience of the therapy or procedure. Part of helping our parents consistently make smart choices involves understanding how to weigh the likely pain and disruption against the potential benefits of the decision. Physicians and family members often think in terms of maximizing outcomes, with too little regard for what your parents may have to endure. Most seniors, on the other hand, are happiest when outcomes are *optimized,* because this approach focuses on maintaining quality, and better enables them to enjoy life. The ultimate goal of medical care for elderly and declining adults should not necessarily be to cure illness or extend longevity, but rather, to make day-to-day life better.

A joint replacement to relieve pain and improve mobility makes sense only if the patient has the mental and physical ability to complete adequate physical therapy. Otherwise, they may never walk again, and would be better off avoiding surgery and receiving treatment to manage their pain. In another example, if a senior has elected to forego treatment for abdominal cancer because of advanced age, they probably don't need a mammogram, pap smear or colonoscopy because the decision that this information would affect has already been made. Information is of limited use unless it is being collected in order to make a decision. Consider the value of the information before you accept diagnostic testing for your parent. The test itself may be more traumatic than the possible benefit of the diagnosis.

What I am describing here is known in the medical industry as *palliative care*. It is a patient-centered approach to care that focuses on optimizing quality of life by anticipating, preventing and treating pain and suffering. The palliative care philosophy embraces both patient and family, and addresses physical, emotional, social and spiritual needs. It can be applied to a senior's particular needs and desires and can even be adapted in response to illness or decline. Palliative care ensures that both you and your parent have the knowledge and understanding you need in order to make confident decisions and to consider the prudence of treating symptoms as a responsible alternative to pursuing cures. It respects your parent's dignity and desire to enjoy their life. In other words, it progresses with your parent as they age and decline, and helps them be in control. Palliative care embodies the perspective that the quality of life is sometimes more important to the patient than the quantity of years.

"Just a spoonful of sugar..."

A good friend recently lost his mother, Madeline, to a fatal heart attack. After her initial heart attack three years before, her doctors had prescribed nitroglycerin tablets in case symptoms of heart difficulties returned.

Madeline lived alone and had decided that, in the event of further heart trouble, the wise thing to do would be to take a nitroglycerin tablet and drive herself to the hospital. With this plan in mind, Madeline kept her nitroglycerin prescription in the glove compartment of her car. Her reasoning was that because she planned to drive herself to the hospital, the tablets would be "right there" when she got to her car.

My friend had repeatedly asked his mother if she regularly replaced her nitroglycerin tablets, knowing that the effectiveness of the tablets would decrease after six months. Madeline replied that she was following her doctor's instructions for medicinal replacements. A call to Madeline's pharmacist confirmed her claims. But as it turned out, Madeline's planning literally had one fatal flaw — temperature. The temperature inside Madeline's car regularly exceeded 110 degrees.

When Madeline's body was discovered, it was determined she died from a heart attack. Although she had taken

her medication, the coroner estimated that her dose of
nitroglycerin had lost more than 50 percent of its initial
effectiveness due to prolonged exposure to extreme heat.

For some unfortunate and unknown reason, too many people discount, or simply ignore, the importance of ensuring that medicine is taken appropriately. In the United States, the number one reason for hospitalization and serious illness among the elderly is the improper administration of medicines. According to recent federal government research, 55 percent of elderly Americans are not following physician's orders for medication administration. [4]

I have an acquaintance who once shared with me that her mother, who had been diagnosed with early-stage dementia, was actually giving medications to her seriously ill, but mentally alert father. I couldn't believe it! She even admitted that her mother had stopped giving some of the father's medication because *she* didn't think it was helping him. No wonder taking medications improperly is the number one reason for hospitalization. Proper administration of medicines is essential to your parent's well-being!

But exactly what is *properly*? Various medical professionals and even drug manufacturers can have significantly different opinions as to how medications should be administered in order to produce the best results. Dosage, frequency, time of day and proximity to meal time are factors that can alter a drug's effectiveness, as well as how it impacts your parent's activities.

A particular drug that is commonly used for dementia patients comes with a manufacturer's recommendation that the medication be given before bedtime in order to cut down on the side effect of nausea. The puzzling nature of this recommendation lies in the fact that the effectiveness of the drug peaks four to five hours after the medication is taken (i.e. while they are sleeping). By giving the medicine right after lunch, our practitioners have found that most people do not experience nausea and that the medicine greatly relieves the issues of increased agitation during late afternoon (i.e. while they are active), which is common among dementia patients.

Dosages of all medications should be closely and carefully monitored. In a home setting, one effective step you can take is to help your parents clean out their drawers and cabinets. The goal is to create a complete inventory of all prescribed and over-the-counter medications in the house. You may be very surprised by your findings. While making the inventory, check to see that the print on all prescription packaging is large enough for your parents to read. If necessary, request large print labels from the pharmacy. It may also be prudent to count pills at an opportune time during the course of every visit.

We once had a resident in one of our independent living facilities who couldn't seem to get her blood pressure regulated. The doctor had changed the type and dosage of her medicine several times, yet her problems persisted. I became suspicious when I heard her story and sent a housekeeper in to "help her clean out her drawers and closet." We discovered a large quantity of pills wrapped up in tissue and hidden all over the apartment. There were two obvious dangers. First, she was not taking the medicine she needed. Second, had she suddenly decided to take her medicine, the changed dosage would have probably been well above what was necessary.

Each pharmacist, like every physician, should have emergency contact information for every customer. Periodic reviews of contact information are advisable. If a parent sees this or any other involvement by you as invasive, find a reason that will make them more comfortable. "They need to have me listed on your account in case I ever need to pick up your prescriptions for you." The pharmacist should notify contacts if medications are not picked up, or are called in too frequently. Don't lose sight of the fact that senior adults can become addicted to certain medications just like anyone else.

It is always a good rule-of-thumb to find a dependable pharmacy that you are comfortable with and always use that same pharmacy to obtain your parent's medicines. For safety's sake, I highly recommend that you take the time to sit with your parents and talk with them about the importance of taking their medicines properly. Make a complete list of medications for each parent. Note both the dosage and frequency. The list should also include over-the-counter medications and vitamin supplements. A straightforward and minimally invasive statement might be, "Mom, I was thinking that if anything ever happens to you and you were unable to speak, I don't know that I would be able to tell the doctor what medications you were taking and your full medical history. Let's get a list of your prescriptions from the pharmacy and then add the other things you take." Once this task is completed, it's a good idea to keep the lists in your parents' LIFE Packets. As with any medical information, always keep the packet up-to-date. If this procedure is followed, then anyone who needs this information should know where to find it in the event of an emergency.

A copy of the completed list can then be presented to the pharmacist or physician for review. In many instances there will be a charge for this consultation, but it will be well worth the cost. If concerns or conflicts are discovered during a review, have an in-depth discussion with your parent's physician regarding medications. The physician should be able to educate both you and your parent as to the grave consequences of taking medicines improperly. While there are times when it may be appropriate to discontinue taking certain medications, this should always be an informed decision, and a physician or pharmacist should be contacted immediately.

The key to arriving at good decisions is to ask enough questions, gain enough knowledge, and establish trust in the professionals who administer care and advise your parents regarding health-related issues.

Conversation 4:
Diet and Nutrition

"You are *how* you eat."

*A*rthur had been a widower for six years. He continued
to live in the house he had built in 1958—the year
after he married Louise. Their three children all lived
within an hour's drive and took turns checking on him. The
children kept in touch with Arthur and each other and had
initiated a visiting rotation as he began to lose his hearing
and short term memory.

While the definition of "checking" differed somewhat
among the three children, none of the children was thorough
in monitoring food or medications in the house. Two of
Arthur's three children seldom ventured beyond the living
room, where Arthur spent the majority of his days—in his
recliner and with his faithful springer spaniel. The family
usually gathered at Arthur's house around the holidays.
Other less formal visits took place regularly throughout
the rest of the year.

One Easter Sunday, all three children brought their
families to Arthur's house for dinner. The grandchildren
hunted for Easter eggs, and stories were told. The dinner
featured a traditional ham with scalloped potatoes—Arthur's
favorite. A grand time was had by all, and by 7:00 o' clock,
Arthur was happy to return to his recliner for a "date"
with Angela Lansbury.

A few weeks later, Arthur's daughter Amy came for a Saturday visit. When she asked her dad if he had taken his blood pressure medication that day, he replied, "Not yet. Could you bring me the pills...with a glass of cranberry juice?" Amy grabbed the pills, and opened the refrigerator to get the bottle of juice. To Amy's horror, the remnants of the ham were perched on the top shelf. When she asked Arthur if he was aware that the Easter ham was still in the fridge, he replied, "It's perfectly fine. It's salted."

Upon further investigation, Amy found several food items that had passed their expiration dates. Similar "surprises" awaited Amy in the bathroom closet and medicine cabinet.

Before taking the first of many trash bags out to the curb, Amy stopped and called her sister and brother. Her message was short and pointed, "We have to meet."

The importance of eating nutritious food increases as adults enter the senior years. Physical limitations and health problems often make it difficult for seniors to maintain a healthy diet. Influenced by a number of factors, poor nutrition contributes to health concerns of 15 to 50 percent of seniors in North America. [5] To complicate matters, the symptoms of an unhealthy or insufficient diet such as weight loss, confusion and dizziness are often mistaken for illness or disease.

Always monitor your parent's diet. Failure to get the proper nutrition can lead to serious problems, but changes in eating habits can also be indicative of other issues, as well. Various strategies may be used to bring this topic into a conversation, but be sure to make inquisitive comments, not investigative ones. You can casually engage them by saying, "We went out for Chinese last night. What did you have for dinner?" Or perhaps, "I have been craving some of your biscuits. Have you made any lately?" If anything you learn in the discourse gives you cause for concern, you probably need to begin keeping a closer eye on things. Consider keeping a journal, noting the type, quality and regularity of meals that are prepared and eaten. If you have a parent who lives alone, you should understand that it is common for them to stop cooking or preparing meals altogether. They may snack excessively and lose the desire for full meals. Mealtimes are very much a social experience in our society. We surround ourselves with family, friends and food, and we interact in the process of consuming our meal. Without this social element, it is easy for a person to lose interest in eating or even lose their appetite altogether. Even with programs such as Meals on Wheels, we have seen instances where elderly seniors have stockpiled much of their food simply because they don't *think* they are hungry. They are often *starving* for someone to sit and eat with them.

Another good habit to develop is inspecting the kitchen. A kitchen paints a thousand words, especially the refrigerator. When your parent is present, casually say, "I'm kind of hungry, what do you have to eat?" As you open the refrigerator door, begin to check expiration dates on items like milk, eggs, cheese, mayonnaise and salad dressings. Inspect any carryout containers to see if mold is present. If the parent is not able to keep the refrigerator cleaned out, this is a sign that you need to take action. Schedule a weekly clean-out. Casually make a list of items to replace, and throw away spoiled, expired and molded food. Seniors are very susceptible to food-borne pathogens so it is important that your parent exercise caution when storing food.

While it is important to know the proper steps involving food storage and handling, it is equally important to make sure the kitchen is well-kept. Have they been cooking? If so, are they cleaning up? Determine if they are using good meal preparation techniques. Have you discovered burners that have been left on? Look for scorched dish towels or plastic ware. Although your parents may have thawed roasts on the kitchen counter their entire lives, this is neither safe nor acceptable. Are meats being cooked at temperatures that are high enough? Be sure that necessary supplies are available and are labeled clearly and correctly, especially harsh cleaning agents. Do not use generic containers for chemicals as this is especially dangerous for seniors with declining eyesight and sense of smell. Applying boldly lettered labels to the original manufacturer's container is the best approach.

———————————————

"Clean up your act."

*R*oy was a retired CPA and a member of my church. He was a decorated Korean War veteran. He was also a diabetic. Despite losing part of his left leg to diabetes years earlier, Roy remained fiercely independent and self-sufficient. Every spring he would grab an ancient step ladder from the garage and clean his roof. Every fall neighbors would hear him in his back yard chopping fire wood.

One day family members were contacted by Roy's neighbors who informed them they had to call for an ambulance after he suffered an injury. Roy had been tilling the ground for his garden when he lost his footing and fell. The blades of the tiller had gashed his right leg, causing considerable damage. The deep cuts on Roy's legs were treated and he was hospitalized for two weeks. When Roy returned home, he shut himself off from the world. Efforts to bring food or show any type of attention were met by a bolted door and exclamations of "Go find someone who needs pity."

Roy's wounds would heal—if given a chance. Ultimately, his undoing was directly related to cleanliness. The bandages were not changed frequently, and the sheets on Roy's bed were, in all likelihood, not changed at all. Roy's attempts to remove the last of the stitches worsened some of the wounds. Inevitably, infection set in. By the time doctors *were able to assess the infection and take action, it was too late. Surgeons amputated the leg at the knee.*

───────────────

The most important health advancement in the world during the 20th century was the ability to provide clean water. The benefits of all the medications and medical procedures and devices around the globe *combined* have not saved as many lives as the advancement of clean water systems. This bit of trivia illustrates the importance of combating harmful bacteria. A person's hygiene and the cleanliness of their surroundings can have a significant impact on their overall health. This is also one of the easiest aspects of your parent's lives to evaluate because you can, for the most part, simply observe. Spending time around them and walking through their home can give you a general idea of how well they are doing in this area. Are they maintaining good hygiene? Have you noticed any excessive body or breath odor? Does the shower appear to have been used and cleaned recently? What about bath towels? Are cleaning and bathing supplies available? Clean healthy skin is the first and best line of defense against bacteria. Bathing is the most important activity related to personal hygiene, but be sure your aging parent doesn't overdo it. Not only is bathing every day typically not necessary due to a senior's lack of activity, it is a bad practice. As a person ages, their body becomes less able to produce the oils necessary to moisturize the skin and maintain its elasticity. As a result, seniors are slower to heal and are more susceptible to skin tears. Be sure your parent uses a gentle, moisturizing cleanser and bathes no more than two to three times per week, with sponge baths in between. Also be mindful of your parent's desire to maintain their appearance. Do they visit the salon or barber as often as they used to? Does their hair appear less groomed than normal? Some of these questions may seem very elementary, but they are an important part of being aware of changes in habits. It is frightening and alarming to see what happens in a senior's home without adequate care and oversight. Small things that go undetected for a long period of time can have grave consequences.

A few years ago an 87-year-old woman moved into one of our facilities. We learned that the HVAC and the water heater in her previous home had not worked for more than a year. The temperature inside the home regularly topped 100 degrees in the afternoons. A neighbor who had become aware of the circumstances installed a window air conditioning unit. With her water heater out, there was no way she could bathe or sanitize dishes with hot water. The concerned neighbor was finally able to contact the elderly lady's niece who lived out of town and was able to resolve the situation.

As you observe the general upkeep of the home, watch for indications of things that have been let go for excessive periods of time. Have you noticed spills that have not been wiped up? Do the toilets appear to have been cleaned recently? Is there an excessive accumulation of dust? A habit you also need to be on the lookout for is *hoarding,* which can really be stockpiling large quantities of anything. High volumes of *stuff* lead to clutter, clutter impedes cleaning, and a lack of cleaning...well, you get the picture. If your observations reveal that your parents are consistently unable to keep their home clean, then it is time for some changes. Perhaps family members can set up a cleaning schedule to share in "helping" your parents clean. If deemed necessary and affordable, consider a cleaning service. Also, many churches will have volunteer groups that conduct visitation and perform household activities free of charge. Always be sure that any volunteer or caregiver entering your parent's home is trained in recognizing unsafe and uninhabitable living conditions. They can serve as an additional source of monitoring of your parent's environment and well-being so make sure they are comfortable contacting you with any concerns.

Conversation 6:
Personal Emergency Device

"One fall away from dependence."

*S*teve and Kathy decided to give each other a number of special gifts for their 50th anniversary. One of these gifts turned out to be a "his and hers" set of personal emergency devices. Steve and Kathy were quite active at the time. In fact, they owned and operated a 150-acre peach orchard and worked outside almost every day. Despite these facts, they realized that they were getting older and that falls and other potential health emergencies were more likely to occur at their age.

One summer morning, Steve was pruning trees in the orchard when he heard the neighbor's truck roar up the driveway. Kathy had been in the barn, detaching a brush cutter from a tractor when she had fallen on top of the cutter. She suffered deep lacerations and was bleeding profusely. Fortunately, Kathy and Steve had not only purchased the personal emergency devices, they had made a pact to use them. Kathy had been able to pull her device from a pocket in her coveralls and signal for help.

Emergency responders were able to rush to Kathy's aid within minutes. After spending a few days in the hospital and a few weeks in physical therapy, Kathy was back on the tractor.

_____

Personal emergency devices can be tremendously important life-saving tools in cases of strokes, falls, heart attacks and other traumatic events. They can quickly prove their worth and provide peace of mind. The devices should not, however, be allowed to provide a false sense of security or to become a senior's rationalization for remaining at home under unsafe conditions. Personal emergency devices improve response time to incidents; they do not *prevent* the incidents.

Any time your parent happens to mention difficulty with particular activities or tasks is a good time to bridge this subject. Be prepared to take full advantage of a comment such as, "It sure is harder to get out of that chair than it used to be." Although they may be speaking from a joking perspective, they are acknowledging increased difficulty with basic activities. This opens the door for you to introduce them to the idea of a personal emergency device. People over the age of 65 should not be without some sort of emergency call system, especially those living alone. The systems available today are designed as a wrist or necklace pendant emergency call system. Anyone can fall, but those over 65 are more likely to experience serious injuries and also take longer to recover. A fast recovery is more likely if the person is found in a relatively short period of time. Dehydration will begin immediately, and if the person is without liquids for several hours following an injury, recovery time will be longer. We had an 84-year-old patient who apparently fell in his home. Although he did not break any bones, he could not get up to call for help. His children found him unconscious in his living room. We suspect he had been there for 18 to 24 hours. His kidneys shut down during his hospital stay, and his recovery took weeks instead of hours.

A personal emergency device should be set up for a caregiver to check once each morning and once each evening. If the device is not pressed, then a call will go out for someone to check on the device wearer. If the person wearing the device is frail and elderly, the system should be set to check five or six times per day. It can be set up to call family, friends and/ or neighbors - not just the 911 dispatcher.

"There's no place like home."
(The Greatest Myth of our Parents' Generation)

I was introduced to Bob at a basketball game. Bob confided in me, "I'm trying to get my mom to come out to your place. I brought her out for a tour, but she had a panic attack before we got to the door."

Bob added that his mother suffered from dementia and was using a medicinal patch. A major concern for Bob was that his mother could not be relied upon to self-medicate properly. "Some days she will be wearing three or four patches, other days none."

Another stumbling block was Bob's brother, who was not ready to move her. It turned out that Bob's brother lived two hours away and was not involved in care-taking efforts. Adding to the family friction was the fact that Bob's mother had begun to accuse him of stealing her money. Bob's brother believed the stories at first. I told Bob that such a scenario is quite common. It is amazing how many children get caught up in their parents' delusions and believe stories that are concocted.

As Bob told me more of his mother's condition and symptoms, I told him that it was very dangerous for her to be living alone. I suggested that Bob go on vacation for a week and have his brother take care of her for that period *of time. Bob's uncomfortable response to my proposal was, "Well, I think he is coming around."*

Bob's brother was not coming around. Bob's brother, unless forced to take care of his mother for a week, will never let Bob put her in "one of those homes." The brother lived two hours away, which might as well be 1,000 miles. However, Bob's brother would be the first to blame him when something happened, proclaiming that he should have done something because he lived so close to her.

One of the conversations that must take place is between family members who take responsibility for their loved ones. Sometimes it might be a sister-in-law or granddaughter who shoulders most of the responsibility. I want to urge all of those caregivers to have honest discussions with other family members about the physical and mental health of those under their care. Every caregiver needs a break, and it is only fair that all members of the family take turns, especially if they are going to be involved in the care giving.

When I reflect on raising my children, I often think about how much their needs have expanded as they have developed. Take *space*, for instance. I remember watching them grow from the bassinet to the crib, then the twin bed and on to a double bed. As they develop, their need for space increases significantly.

Conversely, with an aging adult, the need for space begins to decline.

At some point in life, usually in our twenties, we move away from our parents' home and venture out on our own. As life progresses, we typically require more space due to marriage, the growth of a family and the accumulation of what we endearingly call "stuff." Then, in our forties or fifties, we purchase what we expect will be our last home. It's typically the nicest home we have ever owned, maybe even the one we've dreamed of for so long.

Before you engage your parents in a conversation about leaving their dream home, consider things from their perspective. They love their home. It is that special place where so many special memories have been made. But as time has passed, the children have moved away, and perhaps a spouse is now gone. The parent is probably stuck between emotional ties and current tough-to-face realities. They have a fixed income, an accumulation of possessions, bills coming from so many places and the constant demands of upkeep on the home. They start to close off parts of the house, first the extra bedrooms, then the living room. They may not set foot in these rooms for months at a time. They eventually find themselves sleeping in the recliner or eating in bed. These are not just signs of needing less space but can also indicate deeper internal struggles of a senior who is, for the very most part, at home all alone.

In general, too many people believe that the needs of a declining adult are best met if the senior is kept at home as long as possible. In most cases, this couldn't be further from the truth. Beyond the obvious health and safety issues, a senior left at home becomes increasingly isolated. Regardless of age and abilities, all persons need companionship and human touch. A sedentary life at home often results in significantly reduced mental and physical stimulation, which can lead to emotional and bodily breakdowns.

So how and when do we talk with them about living arrangements? Well, the *how* is the biggest challenge; the *when* is the easier part. Like discussions regarding driving limitations, the conversation addressing living options should begin as soon as possible. This allows you to establish a degree of comfort around the subject and will, over the course of time, very likely give you some insight as to how best to proceed. I recommend easing your way into the conversation as much as five years prior to the anticipated need. On average, that means that by the time the parent turns 75 years old, the decisions and plans have already been made as to where they will go when they can't safely live at home.

As we shift our focus back to the *how*, one of the main points to keep in mind is that you need to be compassionate, but firm. Many seniors even try to insist that their children promise to never put them in "one of those homes." Those words should never be allowed in the conversation, and as I touched on in the Preface of this book, we should not make commitments to our parents that are not in their best interest. Besides, this is a closed-minded and selfish request. It's close-minded because they would be much better off in an environment surrounded by caregivers, activities and other residents with whom they could socialize. The request is selfish because what most parents don't consider is that by seeking this promise, they are asking you to dismantle your life in order to coordinate their household and ac-commodate their daily needs. There is no feasible way that members of the *Sandwich Generation* can properly care for all their parents' needs without putting their lives on hold and unnecessarily taking focus away from their children.

Always be prepared to redirect the conversation and know where you need to take it. The questions that need to be answered are: Where do you want to go when the time comes? Would you like to move closer to me, or do you want to stay in your home community? Do you think it may be a good idea if you go ahead and move while you're still fairly independent, or would you rather stay here as long as you can take care of yourself?

The reality is that once senior adults become unable to effectively care for themselves, it is time for them to relocate to a place where all of their needs can be met on a consistent basis. So if circumstances evolve that warrant your immediate intervention, be prepared to say, "It's time to move; we can no longer care for you at home." Remember, you are guiding your parent toward decisions that are in their best interest but that are, nonetheless, probably contrary to the desires and expectations they have fixed in their minds.

Be very mindful of your parent's condition during a hospital visit. While we always maintain hope for full recoveries, periods of hospitalization frequently mark the onset of changes that can affect your parent's ability to function. You may witness a decline in their ability to bathe, dress or administer medications. They will want to go home as soon as they start to feel a little better. After a week or more of daily hospital visits, you will likely be very tired and ready to get things back to normal. When the health and capacities of elderly adults are compromised, they often tend to mask the truth about their ability to care for themselves or may not actually realize the progression of their limitations. We, as loving and hopeful children, can be more vulnerable to wishful thinking when we are exhausted from the stress of a hospitalized parent. The simple truth is that home may no longer be the safe place it once was for your parent.

It's a good idea to seek the professional opinions of doctors and other staff at the hospital or nursing facility concerning what your parent is capable of doing on their own. Therapists and nurses can evaluate functionality and assess limitations, and activities staff and nursing assistants should be able to share detailed insights. Also, consider calling your parent's pastor. Many seniors may be more open discussing certain issues with their pastor. Ask the pastor to casually approach issues with your parent regarding their ability to care for themselves. Are they afraid to live alone? Are they confident they could summon help if they need it?

Once a decision has been made, it is important to have a clear understanding of the options available in order to make quality decisions for your parent. One option that some families consider is for the parent and the family to "consolidate" (i.e. live together). In recent years, multi-generational living has become the exception rather than the rule. This is primarily because families often do not live in close proximity to their parents. Within this lifestyle, children and grandchildren may benefit from having their loved one as part of their household for emotional and financial support. I have also known several families who have added in-law suites to their homes — suites that were, in later years, redesigned as suites for their teenagers. The funds that would have been paid for a retirement home became equity for the children and grandchildren in subsequent years. Along with these benefits come many disadvantages, as well. If both spouses are employed outside the home, the senior would be left home alone during the workday. In other instances the parent(s) are transported back and forth every day between home and an adult day care center. Also, vacations and other travels are more challenging as the parents would likely require special accommodations during the trip or perhaps alternate care at home if they are unable to travel. However, in the latter case, respite care (i.e. short term) is available in many facilities.

Residential services provided at various care facilities are far more common than these multi-generational situations. While each facility sets up services based on the respective state's guidelines (some of which are controlled by federal regulations), I will use Agapé's organization, developed under South Carolina requirements, as a basis to illustrate the differences in a general sense. I will discuss these in more detail in a later section. There are three main residential categories, each with various types of care levels:

Nursing Facility (NF)

This facility provides in-patient services designed for seniors who need some duration of care and oversight by a licensed nurse. You will likely hear it most commonly referred to as a **Skilled Nursing Facility (SNF)** or perhaps simply a **Nursing Center (NC)**. Nursing facilities are typically licensed by the respective state's health department; in South Carolina, skilled nursing facilities are licensed by the Department of Health and Environmental Control (DHEC). Only nursing facilities that are additionally certified under federal regulations can accept Medicare and Medicaid patients. In general, there are two categories of services that can be provided in a nursing facility. Most states allow a facility to provide both types under a single license:

Short Term Rehabilitation: These services are provided to seniors who are receiving therapy subsequent to a hospital stay in order to rehabilitate from a surgery or acute illness. This may include incidents such as joint replacement, heart attack or strokes. The section of a nursing facility where these services are rendered is sometimes referred to as a **Transitional Rehabilitation Center (TRC).** Its goal is to transition patients back to their pre-hospitalization health, with the hope that they can return to their previous place of residence.

Comprehensive Nursing Care: These services are provided to seniors who have one or more chronic issues that require the ongoing care of a licensed nurse. The services provided in this section of a nursing facility are what most people think of when they use the term *nursing home.*

Assisted Living Facility (ALF)

This is a residential care option available to seniors who only need assistance with certain activities of daily living, such as medication administration, ambulating (i.e. moving about), bathing, dressing, eating and toileting. Assisted living is based on a social model, meaning that medical care is not provided by the facility's staff. This level of care is not federally regulated; therefore its guidelines can vary significantly from state to state. In South Carolina, as in several other states, regulations require that an assisted living facility be licensed. The official state regulatory name for an assisted living facility is **Community Residential Care Facility (CRCF)**.

Enhanced Care: This option is available at some assisted living facilities and provides a higher degree of assistance with activities of daily living.

Dementia Care: This option is available at some assisted living facilities and provides a more secure environment and focused assistance for those with memory impairments, such as Alzheimer's disease.

Independent Living: Designed for seniors who are still able to function independently, but may wish to take advantage of certain amenities and conveniences made available by residing at the respective location. These residents are able to come and go at their own discretion. Many seniors choose this option at a point when they are able to make their own decisions and select a location where they wish to live as their needs progress.

In some states, you may also hear the term **Continuing Care Retirement Community (CCRC)**. These entities usually market from the angle that they can care for your parent throughout every stage of life. While some have traditionally provided multiple levels of residential care and services, many have eliminated or are in the process of eliminating the assisted living component. Instead, they are trending toward providing certain in-home services within their independent living areas, often for additional fees and thereby eliminating 24-hour care. One of the main concerns is medication administration.

"Put your money where your *life* is."

A few years ago, I helped a middle-aged couple arrange long term care for the husband's mother, Donna, whose husband died five years earlier. Donna suffered from dementia and had been living alone until falling and breaking her hip, arm and collarbone. It became apparent that she would not be able to return home.

When the family reached this realization, they began to discuss the topic of long term care. Everyone agreed that this was the sensible solution, and Donna's children made plans to tour assisted living facilities in the area. A second, and rather unpleasant, realization hit the family after the first facility tour—Medicare would not pay for assisted living.

The two children turned their attention to an alternative source of funding — the equity in Donna's house. Her late husband had always been the sole financial manager. The balance on the original mortgage was not sizeable; however, a second mortgage had been taken out to repair flood damage. The end result was that there was little equity in the house.

Donna's children had been piecing together plans to pay for college for Donna's five grandchildren. Suddenly, they were in a quandary — "Do we plan for college or do we take care of mom?"

In the midst of the quandary, an old friend of the family stopped by the hospital to check on Donna. She explained the predicament to the friend. Remarkably, Donna's husband had shared financial information with the friend that he had never shared with his own children. After the "Black Monday" stock market crash of 1987, Donna's husband had invested heavily in treasury notes. Donna may have been aware of this fact at one time, but had no recollection of any discussion on the subject.

With the help of the family friend, the two children searched through old financial records and were able to find the matured treasury notes in a box in the attic. The notes were valued at more than $240,000.

Talking about personal finances can be one of the most uncomfortable conversations, especially from your parent's standpoint. It is very common for parents not to have shared their personal financial status with their children, in some cases simply because they do not want them to know these personal details. But it is important that you are aware of this information and know where your parents keep their financial records. What would happen if a parent suddenly became unable to manage their finances? All too often, children are not exposed to their parents' financial status until crisis strikes. Crisis is the worst time to discover financial troubles.

The recurring theme of "begin as early as possible" is probably most applicable to finances. I highly recommend that this conversation begin around the time your parents retire. If the resources are available, encourage them to seek a certified financial planner who can help them identify all of their financial assets such as home, automobiles, stocks, bonds, retirement accounts, life insurance, projection of social security benefits and, of course, cash. The complexities of properly managing financial assets come with the rising cost of living, downturns in investment performance and stagnant income. The financial stability of an aging adult can erode significantly in a short period of time.

The prudent rule of thumb for a senior in relatively good health is to plan out their financial resources to exhaust at the age of 85. In any case, take the necessary measures to ensure that your parents have proactively researched their financial options and that they make their financial planning decisions in a timely manner.

It is also critical to have someone named as your parent's power of attorney. The authorizations of a power of attorney usually go into effect only due to the incapacitation of the assigner. But in the event that your parents suddenly become unable to care for their own well-being, an executed power of attorney enables and legitimizes management of their financial and legal affairs. Later in the book, I will address additional details about various aspects of financing.

"Learning the ABC's and 'D' of Medicare..."

*D*ot and John met at church when she was 55 and he was 70. John's wife had passed away eight months earlier; Dot's husband died the previous year. John's wife always told friends in the town that he was not capable of living alone and that, if she died, he would grab the prettiest and youngest widow in town and marry her. John and Dot were married after dating for six months.

Dot's family insisted on a prenuptial agreement. Her first husband had sold insurance and had purchased life insurance policies that would provide a generous income for Dot if he preceded her in death. John was a retired professor from a small private college. He had earned a small pension, but his Social Security and home were basically his only assets.

Dot and John enjoyed ten years of travel, friends and family before John became incapacitated with Alzheimer's disease. Two years after the initial diagnosis, Dot found that she could no longer care for John at home and began looking for a dementia facility. To her surprise, they did not qualify for any state or federal funds to pay for such care. Dot discovered that she would have to spend the majority of her own assets before John would be eligible for Medicaid. Because they were married, Dot was expected to utilize her resources for his care. With or without a prenuptial *agreement, they were married; each was expected to provide for the care of the other. An attorney advised Dot to divorce John, but her Catholic upbringing would not permit this option. Dot's children would inherit nothing if John lived for very long.*

Dot could have protected her assets had she bought a long term care insurance policy when they married. At the time, John or Dot could have been covered for $500,000 with as little as $2,500 per year in premiums. In the ten years prior to John's Alzheimer's diagnosis, Dot would have spent only $25,000 in premiums — the cost of five months of his care in an assisted living dementia facility.

The Medicare program is one of the most important considerations in the lives of Americans age 65 and older. Unfortunately, many older Americans and their families do not understand how the system works. Hopefully this chapter will explain the program in easy-to-understand terms so that you can have this conversation with your parents. It is important that they understand Medicare's benefits and select the options most suited to their needs.

Contrary to what most people think, some older Americans do not qualify for Medicare coverage, as it is only available to persons who have paid into the program and their spouses. Many older government and railroad employees did not pay into the Medicare system, as they were provided with other types of medical insurance. Small business owners, clergy and farmers are other groups who may never have paid into the program. As early as possible, be sure to check into whether your parent is eligible for Medicare. If not, find out if they are eligible for any other insurance program benefits.

Many older Americans who do qualify for Medicare underestimate their out-of-pocket expenses. In the absence of supplemental insurance or Medicaid, co-payments and other out-of-pocket health expenses can quickly become significant.

The Medicare program is divided into several parts ("A" through "D"), each of which covers different types of medical expenses.

A very simplified overview:

- "Part A": In-patient services
- "Part B": Out-patient services
- "Part C": Combined Parts "A" & "B" (through approved private companies)
- "Part D": Prescription drugs

"Part A" covers inpatient care services, such as hospitalization and short term treatment in nursing facilities, as well as hospice and home health. Most people do not pay a premium for this coverage. There are required co-pays and deductibles associated with this portion of benefits; there are also limitations on the duration of covered services. For example, "Part A" benefits will cover up to 100 days in a nursing facility for certain illnesses or conditions, as long as the patient's health continually improves during the stay. Once the 100-day benefit is exhausted, there must be a break in the patient's stay of at least 60 days in order to qualify for a new 100-day benefit period. Otherwise, the return stay is considered a continuation of the original benefit period. For example, your mother goes into a nursing facility for rehabilitation after a broken hip and stays for 100 days. She then goes home and has a stroke 30 days later. Because she does not have a 60-day break between events, she would not be eligible for additional covered days in the nursing facility. Due to this limitation, your parent should only use the nursing facility benefit as long as it is truly needed. Always look for a facility that provides rehabilitation six or seven days a week to assure that the maximum amount of rehabilitation is received in as short a period of time as is prudent.

If your parent is being discharged from the hospital to a nursing facility, you should choose the place that you would want for permanent placement, should it become necessary. Once they have exhausted their Medicare days, they would be converted to private pay or Medicaid, potentially making it difficult to transfer to a more desirable facility.

"Part B" covers doctors' services and other out-patient care, therapy and some additional in-home services. This portion of Medicare provides payment for medically necessary services and supplies. Most people are required to pay a premium to receive this coverage.

"Part C" of Medicare may be selected instead of Parts "A" & "B." "Part C" covers more or less the same services and supplies as "A & B," but is provided through private insurance companies that are approved by Medicare. Under "Part C", your parent may receive more benefits at a reduced cost. However, there is a downside with this option. It does not allow supplemental insurance to cover deductibles or co-payments. For example, most people on other Medicare plans have a supplemental insurance that covers the co-pay for nursing facility care after the 21st day. The co-pay will approximately match room and board rate for most nursing homes. The co-pay requirement for many "Part C" plans goes into effect after three to ten days.

Medicare's **"Part D"** is the program for prescription drug coverage. This is another portion of the Medicare benefit for which most participants are required to pay a premium. There are some variations in drug coverage among the plan options under "Part D", but all cover medically necessary drugs. Your parent will be able to choose the drug plan best suited for their particular needs.

Medicaid

Through the Medicaid program, federal and state governments provide health insurance for persons of little or no financial means. There are numerous restrictions on program eligibility, but basically an individual must be completely impoverished in order to qualify.

Medicaid is a federal program that is administered at the state level. Each state sets its own Medicaid budget within federally established guidelines and must fund a portion of the benefits. There are significant program differences from state to state due in large part to variations in each state's indigent population. Most states require three months of residency in order to qualify for Medicaid benefits; therefore, it is often difficult to move a nursing facility patient from one state to another. Moving from county to county within the same state can sometimes prove to be challenging.

In general, Medicaid covers the cost of doctors, hospitals and nursing facilities for those who have exhausted their personal resources. If there is a spouse or child in the home, the program allows for retention of some cash assets and the residence.

Medicaid has a low reimbursement rate for service providers, so this often limits the type and scope of services available to its participants. For nursing facility care, some states pay based on the acuity level (i.e. severity/complexity) of the patient's health issues, whereas others simply pay a flat rate, regardless of the services needed. Of course, if you are in a state that does not have an acuity-based fee schedule, then the nursing facilities are less likely to take a patient who has high-level needs.

The number of Medicaid patients a nursing facility can accept is referred to as its *Medicaid beds*. In most states, Medicaid beds are assigned to each certified facility. That means that each facility has a designated number of beds for which it can receive payments by the Medicaid program. Because Medicaid uses a cost-based analysis to determine its portion of the pay rates, it is very challenging for a Medicaid-only facility to be consistently solvent. Therefore, if your parent is on Medicaid, it is wise to look for a facility that also serves private-pay and short term Medicare rehab patients, as these facilities will typically be more fiscally stable. This is extremely important regarding your parent's care, because you wouldn't want them in a facility that is faced with making budget decisions that could adversely affect the quality of care.

If I am to guide you toward making well-informed decisions, then I feel compelled to be forthright in presenting you with as much insight as possible. The reality is this— when nursing facility staff is deciding whether or not to accept a patient, they have numerous considerations. That's right! The decision belongs to the facility staff, and that decision is usually going to rely on two factors — the patient's complexity of health issues and payer source. So in the end, know that Medicaid is a good and necessary means of health insurance for many Americans. If your parents rely on Medicaid, be sure you understand enough about its challenges and limitations to be able to optimize your parents' access to care.

When Crisis Strikes:
Will you be ready?

The night will come. You will get a call from a parent, sibling or friend of the family. Your mother or father has fallen and is being transported to the hospital. Suddenly, your adrenaline starts to flow. Think! What do I do next? You get out of bed and go to the hospital. Or, if you live too far away, you call someone you trust to go to the hospital with your parent. Whatever you do, you know you can't let your parent be at a hospital without assistance. Even if both of your parents are still living, the spouse needs support and comfort. Decisions have to be made, and someone needs to be the source of clear thought and reason. Are your prepared to be your loved one's keeper?

At *that moment*, you will have just become your parent's parent! You now hold the awesome responsibility of making sound decisions on their behalf. When this time comes, you will need to know as much as possible about your parent's circumstances and what to expect. Even if the length of stay in the hospital is short, the parent will be going home weak and in need of additional assistance. Even a healthy person who has been in bed for several days will have difficulty caring for themselves. Also, hospitals will often discourage non-essential activity. Is there a plan in place to accommodate their needs? Is your parent truly ready to return home? The hospital is discharging them. Doesn't that mean they are ready? Probably so, but remember hospitals are paid by diagnoses, not by length of stay. Medicare pays hospitals based on a schedule of diagnosis-related groups (i.e. the patient's medical issues). Are there supplemental services to assist them once they are discharged from the hospital? In many instances yes, but discharging the patient with home health services or to a rehabilitation facility will reduce the hospital's revenues, so they may be less inclined to order these services. Fortunately, hospitals may end up receiving less revenue if a patient is readmitted, thereby creating a system of checks and balances.

The scenario outlined above was a crash course in suddenly coming to *that moment*. Hopefully, the interactions you have with your parents as a result of reading this book will lead to proactive and timely decisions.

My friend Sam recently mentioned that he was concerned about his parents. His mother has some memory issues, and his father has taken a turn for the worse over the last few months. Sam's sister and brother-in-law live next door to the parents and check in on them every day. Sam lives an hour away and sees mom and dad every week or two. His sister is getting ready to have major surgery; she and her husband will not to be able to spend much time with the parents for a few months. His brother lives in town but runs his own business and is not able to help them at all during the day. Sam is concerned about his parents, but is not sure what to do.

Sam is already in the middle of the crisis and really does not know where to turn. I first asked him to get a list of their medications and to determine the date of the last doctor's visit. His mother is already on dementia medication, but the dose is very low. Because she is more confused and anxious than before, I suggested that Sam get his mother to the doctor to check for a urinary tract infection and check the dosage. Sam's father has not been to the doctor in more than a year, and his weakened state signals that he needs to schedule a visit quickly.

I asked Sam to get together with his siblings, even if by phone, and discuss options for various health-related scenarios. Which rehabilitation center would the parents go to in the event of a hospitalization? If mom or dad ends up hospitalized, then what will the children do with the other parent? What if the parents end up needing long term care? Sam and his wife live just three miles from two reputable care facilities. As a result of their discussions, the children decided that if one or both parents should need care services, both parents would go to the town where Sam lives.

While we can't foresee every circumstance, the key is to possess enough knowledge to make sound decisions. It is your responsibility to step in and help with those decisions, even though they will be some of the most difficult decisions you will have to make. If you have learned all that you can, and if you have had *The Nine Conversations*, your decisions will be much clearer because you, along with your parents, will have made the necessary preparations.

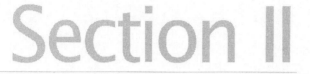

Section II

Residential and Care Options

Making Smart Choices

Now that you understand the concept of *The Nine Conversations*, you will be better prepared to make smart choices on behalf of your parent. At this point, we can turn our attention to the information you will need to know in order to actually implement the decisions you've made with your parent as the result of these conversations.

When choosing a facility for your parent, please do not fall prey to the *convenience factor*. A couple of years ago, I had some close friends who sold their beloved dream home in order to move into a better school district for their children. A new school had been built near the subdivision where they had relocated, and they wanted the highest quality education possible for their kids. Ironically, this same couple is now looking to relocate the husband's mother to another assisted living facility because it will be closer and more convenient to their new house.

Does anybody see the problem here? This is not uncommon. We make what is typically life's biggest investment, move our entire household and often end up with a much longer daily commute to work in order to get closer to the best schools. Then we make decisions on where we "stick" Mom based simply on how convenient the location is to our daily routines. Now, by no means is this comparison meant to suggest that anyone lessen consideration for the well-being of their children; however, it does suggest that you research and give serious thought to where your parent can get the best care.

I recently attended homecoming at a church I had served many years ago. The small town has one nursing facility and one assisted living facility. During my visit, several persons plead with me to bring Agapé services to their town. They were desperate for access to quality care for their loved ones. I listened to numerous disheartening stories about the local facilities. My question to them was, "Why would you leave your loved one in those places? Why not move them to another facility, even if it is out of town?" When I repeatedly heard responses that pointed toward convenience, I was truly frustrated. A thought occurred to me and I turned to ask one lady, "Where did you buy the dress you're wearing?" She halted her answer almost before she started speaking. She suddenly realized the point I was making. You see, I knew the closest town of any size was almost an hour away, rather inconvenient by most people's standards. Yet, she thought nothing of making that drive to get the clothes she wanted. The factors that make it difficult for you to visit your loved one are considerations that may legitimately affect your placement decision. Do not let your reasoning be left simply to convenience. I don't know anyone who even chooses a dry cleaner based solely on convenience. The truth is that convenience is relative to the effort that each of us is willing to make. What I want you to understand from these examples is that what you may consider to be an inconvenient location may, in fact, render the highest quality care for your parent. There *is* a difference in service quality among long term care facilities. Most people, unfortunately, are not familiar with long term care facilities and do realize this; however, it is your responsibility, as your parent's keeper, to ensure that they are placed in a facility that best meets their overall needs.

It is difficult to design a standard regarding care for senior adults due to differing financial circumstances. As we explore care options in this section, I will focus on the "middle class," which describes the majority of Americans and typically includes those who will most likely choose to move into a senior care environment once they are no longer able to care for themselves at home. Also, I will again be describing facility and care services as they exist under current South Carolina regulations.

Nursing Care and Rehabilitation Services

When dining out, it is always reassuring to see a health department rating of "A" posted on the establishment's door. While this rating should be an important consideration when choosing a restaurant, it provides absolutely no indication or guarantee regarding the taste of the food that will be served. Can a top-rated restaurant serve completely unappetizing food? Absolutely, and we have all experienced it. The key to knowing what any grading system tells us lies in understanding what is being graded. The government grading of a food establishment is based on sanitation indicators such as temperatures of refrigerators, freezers and prepared food, and the cleanliness of the facility. While all of these factors are extremely important, they do not affect aspects by which most people judge a restaurant — taste and nutritional value. McDonald's restaurants seem always seem to have an "A" rating, yet the documentary Super Size Me showed how one individual gained 24 pounds in 30 days after eating at McDonald's every day.[6] The point is that it takes a lot more information and consideration than just an "A" on the door to determine that a restaurant is a good place to eat.

Nursing facilities are graded by a similar method. Government teams inspect nursing facilities once or twice a year. The intention is that quality of care is measured and rated by the documentation found in the records and a review of policies and procedures. While a "good" review may show desired documentation and processes, it does not necessarily point to true quality of health indicators. The review primarily seeks to ensure that certain minimum system requirements are met. While this is an important and necessary measure, it should not be the sole determinant in choosing a place for your parent to live. For example, a nursing facility is not graded on the amount of time physicians and or nurse practitioners spend with residents in the facility. So, while a nursing facility is required to have a doctor see each resident every 60 days, there is nothing in the inspection or the grade that would reveal that some residents might benefit significantly from more frequent visits. A sizable percentage of nursing facility residents are admitted for short term rehabilitation following surgery or an acute illness. Yet, the statistics monitored and maintained by government agencies do not grade or give consideration to a facility's success in returning residents to their pre-hospitalization levels of health. Although Medicare-certified nursing facilities are required to provide a rehabilitation program and to screen residents for rehab potential, there is significant variation in the effectiveness of these programs.

Understanding the Medicare system and the respective roles of hospitals, nursing facilities and therapy services is a key component of obtaining the healthiest, fastest and most cost-effective recovery for your parent. As I mentioned earlier in the book, Medicare pays hospitals based on the patient's medical issues rather than length of stay. This means hospitals are paid basically the same amount for treating a patient for four days as they are for ten days, so it makes sense for hospitals to discharge patients as quickly as possible. In contrast, nursing facilities are reimbursed for rehabilitative services based on the number of days the patient receives treatment, provided that ongoing improvement is documented. For hospitals, the primary deterrent against a practice of discharging patients prematurely lies in financial penalties. Hospitals are penalized if patients are readmitted for the same diagnoses within a certain window of time. This is where the right decisions regarding the transition period between hospital and home make sense for everyone. Readmission within 30 days is more likely for seniors who are not discharged to a nursing facility for rehabilitation. [7] A short term rehabilitative stay in a good nursing facility provides much needed therapy and greatly reduces the likelihood of hospital readmission. Because the average daily rates in a nursing facility are a fraction of those of a hospital, this saves the Medicare program thousands of dollars.

As long as your parent has been in the hospital for a minimum of three nights, Medicare will usually pay for in-patient care at a nursing facility, as well as physical, occupational and speech therapies. Be certain that your parent's 100-day Medicare benefit is not exhausted unnecessarily. This means it is extremely important to find a facility that manages care from the patient's perspective. If not, the facility may benefit financially, either directly or indirectly, at the expense of the patient. A facility can actually increase its revenues by prolonging care through its normal practices. For example, if a facility offers rehab five days a week, as opposed to six, the result may be a lengthened recovery time. Even though the facility will likely receive a lower *daily* payment, it can receive more reimbursement overall, as the lengthened recovery period allows the facility to bill for more days. The further the recovery time is unnecessarily extended, the greater the likelihood that your parent's Medicare benefits may be exhausted. Unfortunately, under current guidelines, the government still does not consider the speed of recovery as a criterion of quality in a nursing facility. Also, government surveys do not effectively evaluate the cause and effect relationship between frequency of rehab and length of stay. Even though the first visit to a nursing facility is typically for short term rehabilitation, very few government survey indicators focus on the importance of a quality therapy program. Nonetheless, the length of stay will often be shorter at a good facility, as your parent's rehabilitation will be faster due to more intense therapy.

Home health care can sometimes be a viable option to continue rehab and nursing therapies; however, Medicare will only pay for two to three visits per week. When taking into account this reduced degree and intensity of rehabilitative services in comparison to an in-patient setting, I would consider home health a great option *following* a nursing facility stay.

Rehabilitative therapy continues to gain more appreciation as an effective method of treatment and recovery. When coping with an issue that involves the need for short term rehabilitation, it is important that you understand that the transition period between a hospital stay and the return home can be critical in determining the degree of your parent's recovery. For this reason, I highly recommend that you become familiar with the programs and philosophies of prospective hospitals and nursing facilities in order to ascertain the quickest, safest and most cost-effective recovery plan for your loved one.

When researching rehabilitation services in a nursing facility, arm yourself with the right questions to determine each facility's maximum rehabilitation potential:

1. Is the facility Medicare-certified, and are its rehabilitative services provided under Medicare Part "A?" This will ensure that your parent's Medicare benefits are accepted.

2. Is therapy provided at least 6 days per week? While your parent may not necessarily require rehab every day, having weekend therapy available increases the likelihood that they will receive the weekly maximum of rehabilitation minutes allowed by Medicare.

3. Does the facility offer *split therapy*? This means your parent can receive occupational therapy in one session, take a break, and then receive physical therapy in a subsequent session. Often times, a senior undergoing rehabilitation may not be able to endure multiple hours of continuous therapy. By providing split therapy, seniors benefit from

recovery time rather than missing out on the much needed care.

4. What specific qualifications does the nursing staff have related to your parent's particular needs? For example, if your parent needs wound care, does the facility have experience with wound vacuums?

5. What is the average length of stay at the facility for patients who share your parent's diagnosis? A shorter length of stay can sometimes indicate better quality of care. Be leery of facilities that maximize the use of Medicare days as a practice.

6. Is this the best facility to serve your parent long term in the event that their inability to recovery does not allow them to return home? If this is the case, it is far more difficult to relocate your parent to a different facility than to have their status reassigned within the same facility.

Chapter 11:
Assisted Living

Just as its name implies, assisted living is based on non-clinical assistance rather than the provision of medical care. There are some clear and defining differences between assisted living and the clinical environment you find in a nursing facility. For example, in South Carolina, an assisted living facility is authorized to provide assistance with the activities of daily living, such as bathing, dressing, eating, toileting and moving about. Staff in an assisted living facility are allowed to provide medication administration, but cannot dispense medications. They can follow a doctor's orders, but they are not allowed to interpret them. The ultimate medical authority for any resident is their chosen physician, not a facility staff member.

While most assisted living facilities in South Carolina accept only private payment, the state does offer a program called Optional State Supplement. This state-funded program provides very limited benefits. However, few assisted living facilities participate in this program due to these limited benefits. (See the Financial Planning section for additional information regarding payment strategies.)

Fee Structures and Assessments

First of all, it is important that you understand how fee schedules are typically structured in assisted living. In most cases, the base rate is just the beginning. This is not as bad as it may sound, because if you are paying only a "flat rate," you are probably subsidizing the care of other patients. The most fair and reasonable system of charges is one that most accurately reflects the actual services your parent needs. Most assisted living facilities add care service charges to a base rate to determine a resident's monthly fee. This is usually administered either by incremental *service levels* or *care points*.

Service level charges group a number of services together such as bathing, medication monitoring and incontinency. A monthly charge is assessed to the resident for each *service level* that contains a service needed by the resident. Be mindful that under this structure, your parent can be charged for an entire level even if they only require one service within that grouping. *Service level* charges can typically range from around $150 to $1,500 per month. While most facilities have three or four levels, some have as many as seven different levels of charges.

The *care points* system, on the other hand, allows for the greatest degree of flexibility and personalization when formulating the fee structure. Under this system, points are assigned to the resident only for the services they need. A *care points* charge is then calculated based on those needed services. These charges can typically range from around two dollars per point per day to five dollars per point per day. With this approach, your parent will be charged based on their particular needs.

Both *care points* and *service levels* are determined by assessing the extent and scope of the resident's needs for assistance. As you are researching assisted living facilities, it is important to determine when, how often and by whom assessments are done. Many companies do not perform an assessment until 14 or even 30 days after the resident moves into the facility. This means the initial monthly price quoted for your parent may be significantly underestimated, as they may require more care than could be determined without a full assessment. If this is the case, additional charges would be added to your parent's monthly fee. Subsequent reassessments under the *service level* system could easily mean the addition of several hundred dollars if an additional level is added, whereas the addition of a point may result in less than $100 more per month.

You should always ask questions regarding when and how often the facility's rates are subject to change and whether the facility's administrator helps determine those changes. Many facilities are owned by large publicly held corporations where rates are determined based on corporate profits. Rates in these companies are often determined by boards or officers who have no real understanding of the economic conditions in the local area. Fees for many of these chain facilities increase at rates in excess of inflation in most markets. It's a good idea to ask for the facility's recent rate change letters. Also, beware of rate manipulation tactics. Understanding rate structures and charges is difficult enough without having to differentiate between truth and trickery. For instance, a facility may attract a new resident with a rate based on a low assessment level. Then a month or two later, notification may be received that the parent's rates are going up due to increased care needs. While no system is perfect, it is important to ensure that the facility is providing a good-faith depiction of the expected cost of your parent's care services. Ask about the likelihood of rate increases due to changes in your parent's conditions and have them explain how that process works.

Staffing Levels

Staffing levels have one of the most direct effects on the quality and accessibility of care services. Be sure to inquire as to whether the facility has a predetermined method to calculate staffing needs. If so, make sure the method takes resident assessments into account, as the higher the overall assessed needs, the more staff will be required to provide for those needs. Staffing needs should be driven by both census and assessments. Unfortunately, some facilities will continue to assess people at higher levels without making adjustments in staffing to accommodate the additional needs. Ask how the facility's staffing practices compare to regulatory requirements.

Caregivers, Nurses and Medical Practitioners

While caregivers in assisted living may be trained to collect information and report various situations, such as blood pressure monitoring, they are not trained to make judgments regarding care associated with their observations. The caregivers can only record that information for use by qualified medical personnel. Very few assisted living caregivers are licensed nurses. Even the ones who are licensed are not allowed to provide skilled nursing care within an assisted living facility. Under the best circumstances, some assisted living facilities do employ licensed nurses in order to provide a higher level of oversight and training for their caregiver staff. Because assisted living is not regulated by medical standards and nurses are not allowed to practice under an assisted living license, the execution of physician orders by assisted living facility staff is limited to "medication administration." If a facility you are considering has a nurse on staff, find out how many hours a week the nurse works and if they are on call for emergencies. Be aware of assisted living facilities that advertise a "full-time" staff nurse. Inquire as to whether the full-time work of the nurse in question takes place at that particular facility, or at multiple locations.

Two of the most important questions to be answered are — Who will be involved in managing the care of your loved one, and how can you be sure they will get what they need? The answers should identify both facility and non-facility personnel, as well as how to gain access to these resources. If your parent is moving to a facility in a different town and is leaving behind doctors and other health professionals, then it is important to find a facility that has access to, or will assist in finding, new doctors in the area. Finding out if and when a doctor or nurse practitioner visits the facility is an important piece of information. The more a senior declines, the more important it is to find a facility that has a dependable working relationship with physicians.

It is very important to realize that while physician services may be available at some assisted living facilities, these personnel are not employed by that facility. For example, our physician services are made available to residents through a separate company, just as they would be if a physician were to conduct a visit to your parent's residence. Where on-site practitioner care services are available, it is the resident's right to choose whether or not they wish to utilize these services. Selecting a physician is a very important and personal decision. Electing to utilize on-site physician services can result in several benefits and conveniences to you and your parent. Your parent would not have to leave the premises for most primary care visits or spend extensive time in a waiting room to see a practitioner nor would you be burdened with coordinating off-site visits and possibly having to pay for someone to sit with your parent. The use of on-site services also eliminates your having to coordinate communications between an off-site doctor's office and the facility staff regarding prescriptions, medication orders and records. The convenient access also better enables your parent to be seen by a medical provider on a regular basis, thereby keeping a closer watch on issues as they develop. In addition, having services on-site reduces the risk of falling en route. In order to ensure that providers stay abreast of your parent's conditions, they will typically want to see them at least once every three months and after any consultations or care by outside specialists. Even if your parent wishes to continue seeing their current physician, most on-site services should assist in their medical care by coordinating with other medical providers regarding care management, orders and records administration.

Pharmacy and Drug Administration

Qualified care givers dispense medications in assisted living facilities. It is important to make sure that a nurse and/or pharmacist is monitoring the records and training the staff in medication administration. You should feel confident that the staff who administer medications to your parent have a solid understanding of the importance of this process and that they have access to the proper advisors should questions or issues arise.

Occupancy Rates

Find out how many beds the facility is licensed for, as well as how many beds are currently occupied. Licensing is based on the number of beds a facility can fill, not the number of rooms. Some facilities will present a shared room as a private room when occupancy rates are low. However, once occupancy levels recover, it is probable that the facility will be looking for a way to add an additional person to that room. Be sure to ask whether the room you are considering is a private room or a shared room.

If the facility is not full or close to being full, be sure to ask why. Even though a facility at full capacity is usually a sign that things are running smoothly, there may very well be legitimate reasons for vacancies at a quality facility. For instance, a new facility may have been built in the area, heightening competition. In any case, asking the right questions will usually reveal some valuable information.

Ownership and Administration

Find out who owns the facility and how many other facilities the company owns. Most of the larger chain companies are operated by management teams outside of the state. This means the decision makers may not be familiar with the demographics and regulations in your particular area. Ask how long the administrator has been with the company and how long the former administrator was there. Good administrators are hard to find; be leery of high employee turnover rates, especially in the administrator's position.

Pray, Decide, Act

Contemplating the difficult decisions and assessing the various care options for your loved one can be an anxious, trying, yet reassuring process. While fancy chandeliers, big fireplaces and tablecloths all make favorable impressions, your parent won't truly be able to judge how good a fit a facility is until they've actually lived there. Find out about the reputation of the facility. Ask healthcare professionals, clergy and regulatory officials to give you their earnest opinion of the facilities being considered. Asking family, friends and neighbors to pray about these challenges will go far in revealing the answers and comfort you seek.

Once a decision has been made, don't prolong the process. Many families will make the decision in October but will want to wait until after Christmas to move their parent into the facility. Over the years, we have found that a large percentage of these people do not follow through on their decision, and too often the procrastination affects the well-being of their loved one. Something inevitably happens prior to the move, be it a fall or simply the stress and anxiety of anticipating the move, and all too often, the parent winds up in the hospital. So once you decide, go ahead and make the move. After all, you can always take them home for the holidays.

Chapter 12:
Independent Living

Independent living options vary from free-standing homes located in a variety of retirement community settings, to patio homes, to apartments incorporated into assisted living campuses. With regard to some of the upscale communities, be mindful of what your parent receives in exchange for what are often lofty buy-in fees. It is likely that your parent may be purchasing the "right to live in," rather than actual ownership of the real property. In such a case, it is common to have a guaranteed percentage return on the investment, but that may be dependent upon the owning company's remaining fiscally sound and retaining title to the property. Be sure to have contracts carefully reviewed by a real estate attorney before committing your loved one's life savings.

There are also more moderate approaches to independent living options that maintain freedom for seniors but offer additional services and high-quality amenities. For instance, Agapé offers affordable patio home communities that provide seniors with downsized residences. Purchasers hold title to these units, which include a convenient single-payment system for utilities, and access to a variety of other services. These patio homes carry a guaranteed buyback option, and our real estate company has been able to assist buyers with some very innovative transactions. (See Chapter 21)

Some assisted living communities offer independent living options. When comparing independent living facilities, check to see if the units are licensed for assisted living. The inherent value here is that the occupants of such units will be able to transition to assisted living without facing the stress of moving.

Regardless of the choice you make on behalf of your loved one, be sure to do your research and gain a clear understanding of what they're paying for when the check is written.

Chapter 13:
Palliative Care

As mentioned earlier in the book, *palliative care* is a patient-centered approach to care that focuses on optimizing quality of life by anticipating, preventing and treating pain and suffering. It employs a team-oriented approach for persons whose illnesses don't respond to curative treatment. This philosophy of care encompasses physical, emotional, social and spiritual support, collectively embracing the needs of patient and family. By giving full consideration to your parent's dignity and desires, the palliative care approach can allow them to live each day to the fullest extent possible.

Although it was originally linked primarily to hospice, the utilization of palliative care has steadily expanded to a broader group of patients with chronic or life-threatening illnesses. In today's medical terminology, it means much more than just pain management. The goal of palliative care is to manage all the symptoms of a disease, not to cure the disease.

How does palliative care work?

Palliative care utilizes a variety of healthcare professionals, such as physicians, nurses, pharmacists, social workers, pastoral counselors, a variety of therapists and specially trained volunteers. By pooling the expertise of an interdisciplinary team, care activities can focus on the whole person, not just the disease. Each member of the care team can be brought into the process as the patient and family deem necessary. Some want the entire team to be involved as soon as the patient becomes ill, while others wait until comfort, support and quality-of-life are major concerns. Palliative care can be administered in a variety of settings, including doctors' offices, clinics and long term care settings or at home. Additionally, many hospitals are beginning to develop palliative care programs to augment their existing services.

Traditionally, patient care focused primarily on prolonging life, with far less attention directed at the trauma of decline and death as it affects the patient and family. While today's approach continues to take every reasonable measure to preserve life, additional emphasis is now placed on comfort measures and on preparing patient and family to cope with the process of death.

Under the old concept, as illustrated in *figure 1*, the patient did not benefit from palliative care services until the late stages of illness, often only when death was imminent. Today, as shown in *figure 2*, palliative services begin early in the illness and are elevated as the condition progresses, well before hospice care would be appropriate. In addition, bereavement services are provided several months beyond the patient's death to comfort and assist family.

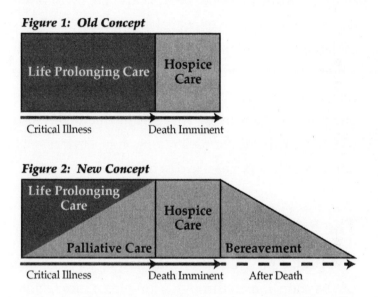

Figure 1: Old Concept

Life Prolonging Care

Hospice Care

Critical Illness

Death Imminent

Figure 2: New Concept

Life Prolonging Care

Hospice Care

Palliative Care

Bereavement

Critical Illness

Death Imminent

After Death

In most cases, a physician or practitioner will be assigned to oversee the palliative care program and coordinate the team members involved in a patient's care. Patients may keep their primary care physician, but the palliative physician or practitioner should coordinate services.

Palliative care is not a hospice program, so utilizing palliative care services does not mean that a patient has to forego curative treatment. Many patients who choose palliative care may also undergo life-extending procedures and therapies.

In some cases, a patient can be eligible for palliative care while on home health care. This will often depend on the resources available and the willingness of the care providers. At Agapé, we can partner with a home health agency in an assisted living or home setting to concurrently care for residents who utilize our physician services. This arrangement can also sometimes afford the patient ongoing services once home health services are discontinued.

The Bridge Concept

A bridge program is a collection of services that can be coordinated through a long term care facility or even home health. For instance, at Agapé we utilize medical practitioners and nurses to provide additional expertise in coordinating pain and symptom management. This enables additional care services for residents discharged to us from hospitals. We are also able to activate support services of other palliative care team members. Under this scenario, even when the Medicare "Part A" benefits expire, the patient may still be able to receive certain covered services.

Who pays for a palliative program?

Palliative care services will be billed to Medicare or other insurance carriers. Because reimbursements for the coordination of palliative care do not exist, the extent and continuation of some services may be limited in certain situations.

Why palliative care?

Only 30 percent of hospitals in the United States currently offer palliative care.[8] But as more healthcare organizations buy into the philosophy, overall patient care and satisfaction will, no doubt, improve. Many patients are trapped in medical limbo, forced to choose between comfort and emotional support in a hospice or a chance to keep fighting their illness. Frequent visits to hospitals involve additional layers of unfamiliar care providers with each admission. An important advantage for a multi-faceted senior healthcare organization is that a patient is afforded the opportunity to receive care as a resident in a facility or at the patient's residence. In instances where a patient decides to remain at home, in-patient care may be available when the family simply needs a break.

This type of palliative team approach can respond any time the patient needs attention, with a deliberate goal of keeping your loved one out of the hospital. Whether responding with pain medication or spiritual counseling, the palliative care team remains committed to caring for your loved one in the least restrictive environment possible.

Chapter 14:
Hospice

The Reality of Death: "Last Things First"

In some respects, the first real conversation you need to have with your loved one actually needs to be about their last wishes. While many consider discussions about death to be morbid, having these tough conversations is the responsible thing to do. There are many issues that are better addressed with a clear mind and before your parent encounters the effects of a major illness. Even though this conversation is advisable, it will likely be difficult and tough to navigate. Helping your loved one plan their senior years is much like going on a long trip. You need to know the destination before you start. So unless you confront this challenge, you may never know how your loved one can be at peace as life declines.

Less than two percent of deaths of persons over the age of 65 are accidental. [9] So, if you are willing to engage in this challenging process, you will most likely be able to assist your loved one in properly preparing for their death. While this may not be a comfortable subject, it is certainly a conversation that needs to take place.

I think each of us could benefit from a chance to "get our life in order." God blessed us with nine months to prepare for the birth of our children. I pray that

I have nine months to prepare for my death. Death is the final experience of our earthly lives. No one should be deprived of the opportunity to have some control over their last days. When the time comes, my wish is for my doctor to give me the facts of my illness and inform me that I have nine months to a year left to live. I would ask for a full assessment of my illness and my doctor's best prognosis of how functional I will be during those last months. I would then take full advantage of time with loved ones and see places I have always wanted to see. My plan would be revisited and readjusted over the weeks and months as my condition changed. During this period, I would also plan a grand funeral and celebration of my life — one that reflects peace in knowing it was a wonderful death.

Even for people with terminal illness, most don't know how long they will have to live. Surveys of oncologists regarding life expectancy among their terminal patients show "substantial variability both within and between doctors" with "significant inaccuracy, imprecision and inconsistency."[10] How do we get things in order? We have to plan ahead.

A few years ago, an acquaintance of mine who owned his own business was diagnosed with a life-threatening illness at the age of 57. He was told that treatment could begin, but there was a strong chance that he might die within the next six months. The man went to his lawyer to make sure that his estate would be in order after his death. He found out much needed to be done in order to clear the estate so that the family would not be taxed to the point of losing the business. A couple of months later, the man decided to get a second opinion and found that his condition had been misdiagnosed and that he was not going to die. Tragically, three months later the man died in a car accident. However, his family followed the plans regarding his business and estate that he had already laid out, and they were able to sustain a very prosperous business that continues to help thousands of people.

Ironically, I knew another man in the same business and close in age, who died of a massive heart attack. A short time after his death, the bank informed his 27-year-old son that it was calling in the notes on his father's business loans. This family's business no longer exists.

When you have this conversation with your parent, there are certain key issues that you need to address specifically, such as questions regarding life-sustaining measures. This part of the conversation should be focused on quality of life measures. The person who may ultimately make any life-ending decisions should be close enough to your loved one to understand them and strong enough to be able to say, "It's time to let go." This will not be a decision based on how old they are or which life-supporting measures to choose to maintain; there's no checklist that will tell you when the time has come. This will be an emotional decision that must be based on the dying person's desires and made in the spirit of compassion.

In addition to honoring the wishes of the dying loved one, there are also many practical considerations regarding end-of-life care options. This is where a clear understanding of the benefits of hospice can make a tremendous difference.

Hospice is a care program developed for persons who are expected to live no more than six months. Hospice includes the services of nurses, social workers, certified nursing assistants and chaplains as well as the provision of certain medicines and supplies. The program also allows for extended services during episodes of excessive discomfort.

The number one quality indicator for end-of-life care is the ability to understand the dying process, as this eliminates the mystery and fear of death. This is one of the greatest contributions of a good hospice care team. I believe the more time a person has with the knowledge that their death is at hand, the better. Even though some people say, "I really do not want to know," knowledge is power and most of us want to have some power and control, even over the manner in which our death takes place. One study found that of 9,000 hospital admissions for life-threatening illness, 50 percent died within six months; 50 percent complained of severe pain throughout most of their illness; and 38 percent died in ICU, having spent an average of 10 days there. [11] In all my years as a pastor and a healthcare professional, I never heard anyone say, "In ICU and on a ventilator, that's the way I want to go." This is the void that hospice can fill. Because many people do not understand the process of death, many fail to embrace the benefits of hospice services. Even when they do, it is often in the latter stages of the dying process. Always keep in mind, physicians take oaths to sustain life and health, so many of them may be hesitant to utilize hospice to the fullest extent of its benefits. Some view it as "giving up too soon" and can unfortunately lose sight of the patient's best interest. Emotionally, most patients want to achieve a sense of control, to relieve burdens on family members and strengthen relationships with their loved ones. Physically, they also need pain and symptom control and want to avoid prolonging the dying process. Spiritually, they want to be at peace with themselves and with God. We have to recognize that death is part of life's cycle.

The Medicare benefit for hospice was established to make appropriate end-of-life care possible. Unfortunately, hospice is one of the most under-utilized Medicare services, with only about 20 percent of Americans receiving hospice care in their final days.[12] While awareness of the program is growing rapidly, hospice has a long way to go before it reaches the potential of providing end-of-life care for all who are in need.

Hospice services are provided under the Medicare program and are paid for through a capped daily rate, which varies from county to county within each state. Under a capped rate system, Medicare will pay the same daily rate for routine care regardless of the services necessary for a patient. If a patient receives services soon after a terminal diagnosis, they may require only limited services during the first few weeks of care. As their condition worsens, the patient will receive a higher degree of services. Some consider the daily rate to be excessive; however, rates are based on the average cost and extent of care in the area. Hospice provides all applicable services related to the patient's diagnosis. Medicare will allow patients to be on hospice provided they meet specific requirements, the most important of which is a medical prognosis of six months (or less) to live.

The majority of money spent by Medicare covers health expenses during the last six months of life. Many Medicare recipients spend their last months of life in and out of hospitals, costing hundreds of thousands of dollars. If a diagnosis of terminal illness is made relatively early, the cost-effective choice is hospice.

Hospice employees seek to educate patients and families about a variety of issues. Hospice professionals are trained in many disciplines in order to take care of the patient physically, mentally, socially and spiritually. And a little-known aspect of hospice care is that it provides ongoing support to the family for a full year after their loved one has passed.

Information gathered from family members whose loved ones died without hospice care revealed that 78 percent felt that they did not have enough contact with the doctor; 51 percent did not receive enough emotional support; and 50 percent indicated that there was not enough information of what to expect during the dying process. [13] Surveys have indicated that the more money spent on healthcare in the final days of life, the lower the satisfaction results. Those whose loved ones were treated in high-intensity hospital environments reported lower quality of emotional support, decision-making information and respect. In other words, the more hospitals tried to do for the dying patient, the greater the family's dissatisfaction with the experience.

If and when a family's comfort zone and level of understanding are jeopardized, situations quickly become critical. At such times, practical support and assistance, as well as trustworthy information and advice, are all of paramount importance.

Quality care is what a good hospice organization is really about. The reimbursement system helps take the focus away from money, better ensuring that patients are treated in a fair and equitable manner and that they receive the care and compassion they need and deserve.

_____

Isolation, unsafe living conditions and limited social contact are just a few of the problems facing seniors today as they struggle to stay in their homes. In some cases, seniors may be physically functional, yet unable to cope with the burden of maintaining a residence. Unfortunately, it frequently takes a crisis, such as a fall, to realize that a loved one can no longer live safely at home alone. That is unfortunate because these kinds of setbacks usually end up robbing the senior of what should have been more quality living time. Many seniors will, nonetheless, selfishly wish to remain in their own homes even when their abilities decline, and this comes at a great cost for those who must care for them.

Home Care Services

Staying home may be an option as long as the senior or someone living in the home is capable of making day-to-day decisions regarding care. If someone in the home is mentally alert, they should be able to hire, fire and direct the necessary assistants and caregivers.

Home care service companies provide basic assistance with activities of daily living such as bathing, dressing, cooking and light housekeeping and generally charge a relatively high hourly rate in relation to the services provided. They generally charge about two times the typical rate for a caregiver. Be sure to inquire specifically as to the caregiver's qualifications as they may not be allowed to administer medications. Many states have made it illegal for anyone other than a family member or qualified medical personnel to administer medication in a home setting. Mistakes involving medication administration are often made by family members or other caregivers. For example, a daughter takes mom to a doctor's appointment, and the doctor changes the type of blood pressure medication. That night, the sitter comes in and sees two prescriptions on the table. The labels on the two bottles are different, but both labels instruct the patient to take four times daily. If the sitter were to administer both medications, a likely result could be a sudden drop in blood pressure and a resulting loss of consciousness.

There are a few government programs for the indigent that do provide home care service. A key requirement is that the patient qualify for skilled nursing services, which means they shouldn't be at home. Such programs and benefits are very limited.

Because there is no significant government funding involved in home care services, most states do not require a license to run these agencies; therefore, there is no oversight by the state. As a result, there are significant variations in quality of care. Also, any situation where an elderly adult has service providers entering their home also gives rise to concerns of vulnerability. An elderly lady moved into one of our assisted living facilities after her daughter discovered she had signed over the title of her vehicle to the sitter. The sitter had manipulated the mother by telling her that her automobile insurance might not cover the sitter when she was driving because it was not in her name. Of course, by the time the daughter found out, the sitter had vanished.

The financial costs of home care services and reliability issues with sitters often lead people to seek other care options.

Home Health Agencies

Home health care (unlike home care services explained in the previous section) is provided by agencies authorized to perform certain nursing and therapy services within the patient's home. Home health companies must be licensed and certified, meaning that the state and federal governments establish standards, provide oversight and conduct inspections. These agencies are generally directed by a physician, and services are provided by a licensed nursing and therapy staff. Most home health care is limited in duration as these services are paid for based on diagnosis rather than services rendered. Medicare provides payment for these services under a capped payment system. This means that the home health agencies receive the same amount of compensation no matter how long or how much care is provided. While Medicare provides guidelines for home health care, much discretion is allowed. Most agencies will typically send a licensed nurse to the home twice a week and a nursing aide or home health aide up to three times a week. Because of the capped payment structure, the sooner they can discharge a patient, the greater the profit.

The primary point to recognize here is that home health care is not provided on a daily basis nor does it allow for 24-hour services. In addition, it does not address the concerns of isolation. When a social worker or discharge planner at a hospital states that home health care is available, keep these limitations in mind and be comfortable inquiring about all options available for your loved one.

———————————————————

Section III

Health Issues

The Information You Need

In addition to understanding residential and care options, it is imperative that you are familiar with some of the health issues that commonly affect senior adults. Your ability to anticipate, recognize and prevent these problems can serve to protect their quality of life and wellbeing.

When it comes to managing the health of your loved one, I strongly encourage you to be well-informed and to be directly involved in the decision-making process. Family members should have a strong rapport with any provider caring for their parent, and they should definitely take advantage of every opportunity to meet with their doctors. Although this may prove to be inconvenient at times, it is well worth the effort. Be aware that seniors are not always forthcoming when it comes to their health, as they do not want to burden anyone with their issues. As a result, it is important to speak directly to their various care providers. In a nursing facility, this includes administrators, nursing staff, therapists and doctors. Physicians who provide care in nursing or assisted living facilities should offer consultation appointments with families in order to discuss medical issues.

Too often, in both hospital and nursing facility settings, family members stop by after work and end up talking to health professionals who work second or third shift. While these persons are as competent as other caregivers, they have not had as much firsthand involvement with your parent's care. Keep in mind that first-shift staff typically work from 7:00 a.m. to 3:00 p.m.; the majority of treatment normally takes place during these hours.

Treatment during the transition period after a hospital stay is extremely important, as it relates to your parent's recovery and ability to function. Upon their discharge, the same holds true for the relaying of information regarding their treatment while in the hospital. This information is critical to your parent's ongoing needs and should be accurate and thorough. Please remember that you, as well as a nursing facility, may be limited by the availability of information that hospitals or doctors share if you don't make the extra effort to confirm your under-standings. That's one reason I recommend that you carefully review hospital discharge orders and other information against any dialogue you may have had with the hospital's physicians or other providers. For example, we have had complaints from residents involving dietary restrictions that were incorrectly ordered by a hospital physician. A quick review of dietary orders by a qualified professional can usu-ally clear these mistakes. If a nursing facility has a physician's order for certain dietary restrictions, it must be followed by facility staff.

Even if it means taking some time away from work, be sure to speak with the providers that are most actively involved with your parent's care in order to get the most complete and accurate information possible.

While there are numerous issues that contribute to the decline of a senior's well-being, I want to discuss a few of the more prevalent ones. While these conditions are rather common, they are nonetheless often underestimated and misunderstood. Hopefully the chapters in this section will assist you in gaining a greater awareness of these issues and what can be done to manage their effects.

Chapter 16:
Hip Fracture

The Serious Consequences of Falling

Falling is the number one cause of injury for senior adults. Each year, one in three Americans over the age of 65 will be injured in a fall. [14] Approximately half of those experience multiple falls. [15]

Both the frequency and severity of falling increase with age, as does the difficulty of recovery. Any fracture must be taken seriously, especially one suffered by an older adult. A study based on Medicare records tracked deaths after more than 600,000 hip fracture surgeries from 2000 to 2002. The study underscores the apparent link between aging and fracture-related deaths. Thirty-six percent of those 85 and older died within a year of their injury, compared to 19 percent of those 65 to 74.[16]

While we should take measures to guard against falls such as wearing clothes that do not impede normal movement, wearing slip-resistant shoes, maintaining clear pathways and exercising, it is practically impossible to prevent a fall.

Historically, physical restraints were used to prevent individuals from getting up without assistance. However, increased awareness about the negative effects of this practice, along with the development of safer devices, has significantly decreased the use of traditional restraints. The use of restraints also poses added risks for people who are agitated, as they may nonetheless fall or damage muscles while attempting to escape their restraints. There are potential psychological effects as well; restrained individuals often feel humiliated. They may become depressed, withdrawn or agitated when freedom of movement is denied them. Numerous studies have demonstrated that the risk of serious injury does not increase when physical restraints are replaced with less-restrictive safety measures, and behavior problems usually decrease notably when restraints are removed.

Restraints are sometimes useful and necessary as a temporary measure in providing needed medical treatment such as intravenous medications, specialized feedings, wound care or when other less restrictive measures have failed to provide adequate safety. However, applying physical restraints routinely or for prolonged periods should be avoided. Overuse of restraints can result in increased dependence, incontinence, infection, pressure sores, social isolation, decreased balance and de-conditioning. It is sadly ironic that these same issues are brought on by falls.

Dealing with the issues of falling can be one of the most difficult challenges related to senior care. Spouses and children struggle with guilt when their loved one falls, and are often tormented by the thought, "If only I had done something differently." But the unfortunate truth remains—you simply cannot prevent falls.

A few years back, my wife was reading an article about former president Ronald Reagan, who suffered from Alzheimer's. She looked up as she read the article and exclaimed, "Ronald Reagan fell." I said, "Yes, he has Alzheimer's and falling is a common occurrence with Alzheimer's patients." She exclaimed again, "No! Ronald Reagan fell!" Again, I replied, "Yes." She then explained her disbelief. This former president of the United States was guarded closely by secret service agents and was surrounded by highly-trained caregivers, yet he still fell.

Injury resulting from a fall can contribute a number of other serious health issues. Post-fall care plans that include strategies to reduce pressure ulcers, increase vaccination and treat pneumonia are vital to a senior's recovery after a fall.

Another factor that affects recovery after a fall is response time. The sooner a senior is treated after a fall, the less the likelihood of secondary complications. Personal emergency devices, as discussed in Conversation 6, can prove to be invaluable when falls occur.

Even when a fall does not result in serious injury, it often leads to self-imposed mobility limitations. The fear of falling, which occurs in about half of all seniors, can cause an older individual to lose confidence in their ability to perform activities safely. This fear is associated with functional decline, decreased quality of life, increased depression, and increased risk of falling. Decreased mobility that occurs as a result of injury or psychological trauma, such as the fear of falling, can lead to fall-related complications.

One study revealed that depressed patients were 57 percent more likely to die within two years of a hip fracture than patients who had a positive outlook.[17] Statistically, there was no difference in death rates at the one-year mark, but the cumulative effects of depression were clearly evident after the second year. Even mild depression can slow recovery. As many as half of all seniors who break a hip suffer some symptoms of depression and are more likely to end up in nursing homes. Caregivers who provide extensive rehabilitation and encouragement can greatly assist in recovery.

Delirium — a condition that affects as many as 60 percent of seniors who are hospitalized for hip fracture surgery— can be further complicated by depression. [18] The sudden mental confusion associated with delirium can be triggered by infections, pain and immobility, all of which are common problems after hip surgery. Anesthesia and pain medicines can worsen matters. Hallucinations are usually the initial symptoms, but some patients become withdrawn and sleepy, making delirium difficult to diagnose. The consequences can be severe. Research has shown that hip patients with delirium were nearly three times more likely to die in the first six months after a fall. For patients who survive, symptoms can last for months, and can reduce the effectiveness of rehabilitation.

After the Fall
Topics to Discuss with Your Physician

- Antibiotics. If surgery is required, make sure the surgeon prescribes antibiotics before and immediately after the operation.

- Blood clots. Take anti-clotting drugs, as prescribed.

- Loss of mobility. Discuss the need for appropriate medical equipment.

- Delirium and depression. Discuss warning signs.

- Exercise. Returning to walking as soon after a fall as is deemed safe will improve the chances of full recovery.

- Therapy. Comply fully with all physical therapy and occupational therapy orders.

- Long term follow-up. Seek help from a geriatrician, family doctor or nurse.

The following list reviews recommendations that can help lessen the likelihood of falling for seniors:

- Exercise: Walking is helpful, but strength training offers the most protection. Strengthening muscles can help compensate for weakening bones.

- Improve balance: Balance improving exercises such as Tai Chi can reduce the likelihood and fear of falling.

- Reduce hazards at home: Remove clutter from floors and stairs. Install grab bars in bathrooms and non-slip mats in bathtubs. Improve lighting and install handrails on stairways. Make sure rugs and other floor coverings do not create hazards.

- Dress safely: Avoid loose-fitting clothing. Wear properly-fitting, slip-resistant shoes, not slippers.

- Be mindful of pets and pet leashes.

- Control blood pressure: Many falls are caused by dizziness that can result from low blood pressure or from a rapid drop in blood pressure when attempting to stand up.

- Be aware of side effects of medications: Some medicines affect the mind, such as sleeping pills and anti-anxiety drugs; others, like cortisone, can weaken bones.

- Maintain a healthy diet: Good nutrition is essential for bone and muscle strength, as are Vitamin D and calcium. Monitor for anemia and take iron supplements, if needed.

- Monitor health: Get a bone density test to check for osteoporosis, and get treatment to strengthen bones or prevent bone deterioration.

- Watch for warning signs: Falls that don't cause injury are often warning signs for more serious falls. Seek medical help to identify causes.

- Home assessment. A physical or occupational therapist can inspect the home for potential hazards.

Chapter 17:
Dementia

*D*ementia is a word that is usually associated with loss of memory. Other symptoms include time and place disorientation, depression, poor judgment and loss of initiative. The behavior and personality of dementia patients can undergo drastic changes.

Short term memory is especially problematic for dementia patients. As a result, topics of conversation may be forgotten and repeated frequently, often within a very few minutes. Dementia patients can forget basic things, like how to place a phone call. People who have dementia may put things in the wrong place. They might put a frozen turkey in the linen closet or the out-going mail in the microwave.

The National Institute on Aging sponsored research that shows that older adults who exercise at least three times a week are much less likely to develop dementia than those who are less active.[19] In the early stages of dementia, memory loss is often dismissed as a general sign of aging, but memory loss from dementia often progresses severely and rapidly and can be accompanied by one or more additional symptoms.

Many diseases and events can cause dementia, including Alzheimer's disease and strokes. More than five million Americans have Alzheimer's disease.

That number could triple to 16 million by 2050, as baby boomers join the over-65 age group. [20] An ever-growing variety of drugs has been created to help dementia sufferers. While these drugs cannot cure dementia, they may lessen symptoms or slow down progression of the disease.

Special Care for Dementia

Dementia care is challenging due to family expectations, misinformation, and regulatory issues. One regulatory example involves doorways. Building codes for facilities housing dementia patients require that buildings be evacuated in the event of disasters. The doors can have delayed exit, but cannot be locked. Although exit doors can be alarmed, they must open within 15 seconds of the touch of the panic bar. The regulations make design and staffing extremely important; they also make it virtually impossible to secure a building.

Get Into Their World

During the onset of dementia, patients are usually aware of the fact that they cannot remember and, as a result, can become very agitated and frustrated in conversations. It is very important for caretakers to have patience.

A visit to a dementia unit should be an act of kindness and love, with the intent of making that person's day a little better. The visit must be about the dementia patient, not the person visiting. Expecting or hoping that the dementia patient will remember some event, time, place or person is unrealistic.

A dementia patient might be convinced that the current date is some point in the 1940s and might remember the familiar face of a son as that of her husband or former boyfriend. The patient can enjoy the visit by discussing the war years or remembering cultural events, including music and books from a previous era.

The patient might remember being a young mother and find peace in carrying a doll or might enjoy a kitten or dog that comes to visit. Arranging flowers, pretending to sew, watching old movies or even eating a hamburger and milkshake might be great treats to enjoy as part of a visit from friends and family.

Children are a delight to some dementia patients. For others the unpredictable nature and/or energy level of a child might too much. Don't set your sights on the hope that your demented mother will be glad to see her new great-grandchild. While such an opportunity might be terrific for some patients, others could find such a visit to be a disaster. The key to every visit is to have no expectations for regained memory. Never ask, "Do you know who this is?" That line only creates anxiety and confusion and can lead to a total meltdown.

Alzheimer's disease is just one form of dementia. For the purposes of this book, the word "dementia" will serve as a catch-all for any of a number of memory problems. My first experience with dementia was with Jake, a member of the first church that I served after completing seminary. Jake was 60 years old when I first met him. He lived with his wife, Bessie. Jake had managed plantations all of his life. He was a big man, standing well over 6 feet tall, with a muscular build. In his job, he would arrange hunting and fishing trips for visitors to the plantations. He also made sure that the grounds were well-maintained.

A year before I moved to the area, Jake started forgetting things. At first it was irritating to Bessie; he would go out for bread and milk and return with nothing. Jake would offer excuses when he did not remember things. She asked her friends, and they all laughed at first, joking that it was "all men." One day,

Jake left early to go to the farm and check on things. He usually returned for lunch, but when he had not returned by 3:00 p.m., Bessie called one of the farm hands to look for him. Ellis had worked with "Mr. Jake" for several years. He was loyal and dedicated to the man who gave him work; Ellis also looked after Jake like family. Ellis searched for Jake and, at about 6:00 p.m., returned to the house with him. For the better part of the day, Jake had been bewildered and confused. Ellis found him sitting in his truck, completely disoriented. Jake had become lost on a farm that he had been working for most of his life.

Bessie and Jake began to visit doctors, going from their local physician to several specialists. Tests ruled out almost every possible diagnosis that could have caused the memory lapse: Parkinson's disease, depression, meningitis, epilepsy, Pick disease, stroke, cerebrovascular disease, head trauma, Lyme disease, Lewy Body, prolonged toxin exposure, thyroid disease, vitamin deficiencies, hormonal imbalances (most women suffer with this during menopause) and Wilson disease

After undergoing scores of tests, the diagnosis, through a process of elimination, was Alzheimer's disease. The diagnosis, like almost all Alzheimer's diagnoses, was the result of a process of elimination and was based on signs and symptoms. An autopsy was the only way a definitive diagnosis for Alzheimer's could have been made.

Chapter 18:
Parkinson's Disease

Parkinson's disease is caused by a loss of neurons in the area of the brain that controls motor functions. When this occurs, there is loss of control of movement, which is one of the main symptoms of the disease. Medical science has yet to determine exactly why this occurs.

Parkinson's commonly affects cognitive skills, as seen through symptoms such as loss of decision-making, inability to learn and adapt to change, disorientation, difficulty concentrating and loss of short or long term memory. Persons with Parkinson's also respond slowly to questions and requests. They become dependent, fearful, indecisive and passive. As the disease progresses, they become increasingly dependent on spouses or caregivers.

Contrary to popular belief, not all persons with Parkinson's shake noticeably. The signs and symptoms of the disease are very closely related to other forms of dementia; therefore they are very often misdiagnosed. While the indicators are similar, the medical treatments used for a person who has been diagnosed with Parkinson's are very different from those used for other forms of dementia. Proper diagnosis and treatment can lead to stabilization, or even a reversal, of dementia symptoms.

I have witnessed the repercussions of misdiagnoses on many occasions, but a particular case that comes to mind involved a resident who moved into one of our assisted living facilities. Although the patient used an outside family doctor, Agapé's physician was asked to see the resident one day when he was experiencing an acute episode. The resident was combative and confused and constantly tried to escape. Because our physician had seen many Parkinson's and dementia patients, he was able to recognize the difference in the man's actions and prescribed a Parkinson's medication. Three weeks later, this man was able to move back home with his wife. His confusion was significantly reduced, and he was fortunate and thankful that circumstances caused the intervention of our physician and a correct diagnosis.

Chapter 19:
Urinary Tract Infection

In elderly men and women, bladder muscles progressively weaken over time. This weakening leads to increased residual urine volume, less-efficient bladder emptying and incontinence. Many older adults are not comfortable talking about issues related to their bladders and bowels, so they endure, hoping the problems will subside. If your parent shows signs of confusion, frequent urination, strong urine odor, bloody or cloudy urine, pain or burning with urination and/or pressure in the lower pelvis, a urinary tract infection is a likely culprit.

Interestingly enough, elderly adults with urinary tract infections are sometimes misdiagnosed. An elderly person with a urinary tract infection may suddenly become confused. According to MedScape.com, up to 35 percent of elderly patients with serious infections do not exhibit the hallmark sign of a high fever. [21] This is due to the common inability of an aging immune system to mount a response to infection. As bacteria in urine spread to the blood stream and cross the blood-brain barrier, confusion and other cognitive difficulties can be the end result. Sudden onset of these symptoms should prompt one to investigate a possible urinary tract infection. An elderly person who is experiencing mental difficulties should also be closely monitored for other symptoms of a urinary tract infection.

Section IV

Financial Planning

Why Plan?

Regardless of the decisions you wish to make with your loved one concerning their wellbeing, you have to be ever mindful that all care options will come at a cost. Careful planning in anticipation of these costs is the most effective way to ensure that the best options are available when the time comes.

Calculations by the Vanguard Group based on data from the Society of Actuaries reveal that a 65-year-old single male participant in a retirement plan in 2007 has an average life expectancy of 82.5 years. Within this group, there is a 67 percent probability that a person's life will end between the ages of 74.5 and 90.8 years. [22] Studies published in The New England Journal of Medicine show that more than 40 percent of Americans over the age of 65 will have at least one stay in a nursing facility. [23] Other recent figures indicate that more than half of the average individual's lifetime medical costs are spent during the last year of their life. So what do all of these statistics mean to you? They mean that many people will be living longer lives, and it's going to cost quite a bit of money to pay for their care. In other words, financial planning is a critical component of your parent's future if you want them to have the best care.

Chapter 20:
Long Term Care Insurance

D o your parents have Long Term Care (LTC) insurance? This is a very important question to answer in relation to their financial planning. If not, I would encourage them to explore their options with a long term care insurance agent.

Some financial advisors are of the opinion that long term care insurance may not be a well-suited option for every circumstance, especially when an individual has a low income level and little or no assets. But short of being extremely wealthy, not having long term care insurance can significantly limit a declining senior's access to care options. Because Medicare does not provide a long term care benefit, Medicaid may be the only accessible care option outside the home. Even so, many states, including South Carolina, provide little or no Medicaid coverage for assisted living. This means they would not be able to access the primary Medicaid long term care benefit until their health declined to the point where they qualified for skilled nursing care. This means that they would require 24-hour attention of a licensed nurse. Nearly half of all Americans over the age of 85 need assistance only for activities of daily living. This group would be appropriate only for assisted living and, therefore, would not qualify for the Medicaid benefits available in a nursing facility. If your parent is not able to afford long term care insurance, you may recognize the benefits of subsidizing or even covering the long term care insurance premiums in order to ensure access to suitable long term care.

I bought my first long term care insurance policy at the age of 38. Many people will argue that long term care insurance coverage may be useless by the time it is needed, but that is speculative. It also assumes that policy holders would need the benefits only in their later years. One consideration that people often ignore is the possibility of a debilitating injury at a younger age. Although such injuries are not very common, I once had three residents under the age of 40 in a nursing facility. One of these individuals had fallen from a ladder and severed his spinal cord. Once his health insurance covered the maximum liability, all other expenses were the responsibility of the family, and, unfortunately, he did not have long term care insurance. Eventually, after losing all of his assets, the man applied for Medicaid.

I have been questioned by friends as to why I would need long term care insurance. After all, I'm the CEO of a network of assisted living and nursing facilities. Granted, if I needed care today, I am fortunate enough to have the assets and resources to care for myself and my spouse. But who knows what the next 30 years may bring? It is always a sobering experience to see families forced to make decisions regarding the care of their loved ones based solely on affordability rather than quality.

I have also heard comments like, "I'm not worried. My children will take care of me." It would be nice to think we could count on that, but consider this — we have several residents in our long term care facilities who are more than 100 years old. That means that their children are in their seventies and eighties and are probably not physically able to care for their parents. In many cases, they are not financially able to care for themselves, much less for their parents.

Policies for persons under the age of 40 are very inexpensive because the likelihood of claims is extremely low. The policy I purchased at 38 was for a specific dollar amount, but was good for my lifetime. I continue to fund this policy because it is still very cost-effective. In addition, I have added a second policy to assist in covering today's higher cost of care. The optimum age to buy long term care insurance is from age 45 to age 55. Premiums are less expensive because people generally do not have medical conditions that would make them uninsurable. Individuals who are already past this age bracket should consider buying coverage around age 65.

Some policies contain certain requirements of the service provider, such as 24-hour staffing, an on-call physician and medication supervision. Be sure to look for as much flexibility in coverage as possible. A good policy will cover residency and care in both assisted living and nursing facilities. Try to find a policy that pays when the holder cannot perform two or more activities of daily living. One of these activities should be bathing because virtually all nursing home residents receive help with this activity. Any in-home benefits should cover adult daycare, hospice services and respite care. Keep in mind that as new systems of care emerge, they may not be covered by some existing policies. For example, 15 years ago long term care coverage did not pay for room and board in an assisted living facility. Keep a close eye on the coverage details of the policy and update or supplement as needed.

Purchasing long term care insurance can be difficult for individuals with chronic conditions like diabetes that could prove to be incapacitating over time. Also, persons over the age of 70 are often unable to pass the medical tests required for qualification, or it may simply be cost prohibitive for someone of that age. No matter what the circumstances may suggest, it is always advisable to assist your parent in researching and considering all available options.

Our insurance company recently sold a long term care policy to a woman over the age of 80. With the payment of her first $800 monthly premium, she had $500,000 worth of long term care coverage. She made a very wise investment even though the premium is costly, because she has now protected her financial assets.

Long term care insurance helps protect your assets. Unlike qualifying for Medicaid where the applicant can only have very limited assets and income, purchasing a long term care policy allows the policy holder to retain all their assets as well as any income they may be receiving. In addition, it is a very prudent strategy for anyone wishing to leave an inheritance. It is sometimes possible to purchase a long term care policy that can be excluded from Medicaid considerations. It is always best to consult a certified provider of long term care insurance within your state regarding the most up-to-date information on government programs and insurance guidelines.

The cost of long term care insurance is a considerable obstacle for many Americans. But an insightful comparison of the costs and benefits can be enlightening. Let's say your parent bought a long term care policy with a $1,200 annual premium and paid on it for 20 years. That is a total investment of

$24,000. Today's cost for a private room in a nursing facility ranges somewhere between $200-$260 per day, or about $7,000 a month. Assisted living for a high-level care or Alzheimer's resident can be every bit as expensive, and standard assisted living will run well in excess of $3,000 a month. How many months of care could your parent afford with the $24,000 paid in premiums? It would cover three or four months, maybe six at the most, depending on how their needs progressed — certainly nowhere near as many as the long term care insurance policy would cover.

Reasons to buy LTC Insurance:

- Greater level of independence and care options.

- Reduction of financial and emotional burdens on family members.

- Flexibility to obtain quality care in an appealing location.

- Reduced reliance on government-paid programs.

- Preservation of assets for spouse/children.

- Peace of mind regarding well-being.

Tips for buying LTC Insurance:

- Buy only from top-rated companies (good products come from good companies).

- A.M. Best, Standard & Poor's and Moody's Investors Service all provide ratings.

- Buy inflation protection (inflation can devastate the true value of a policy).

- Buy an appropriate level of coverage (consider income from other sources).

- Consider a Shared Care Rider (combines benefits for use by either spouse).

- Avoid as many other riders as possible circumstances can change overnight).

Chapter 21:
Reverse Mortgages

A home equity conversion mortgage, more commonly known as a reverse mortgage, is a special type of home loan that allows the owner to convert a portion of the equity in their home into one of several cash options or a line of credit. The home equity conversion mortgage program is authorized under the FHA and is available to homeowners 62+ years of age who own their home free and clear (or hold a very low mortgage that must be paid off at closing with loan proceeds) and who occupy the home as a primary residence. Interested persons are required to receive agency-approved counseling before applying. There are some reasonable upfront closing costs, but otherwise, the borrower only has to keep taxes and property insurance current, and pay a very nominal monthly mortgage insurance fee. The reverse mortgage itself does not have to be repaid until the borrower no longer uses the home as their primary residence. When the property is sold, the borrower or the heirs will receive any monies in excess of principal and interest. However, should the mortgage balance be greater than the value of the property, no more will be owed than the value of the property provided it is sold for the purpose of repayment.

The amount of money that can be borrowed depends on the borrower's age, the current interest rate and the lesser of the appraised home value or the applicable FHA mortgage limit. In general, the higher the home value and older the borrower, the higher the loan amount and lower the interest rate. Keep in mind, however, that reverse mortgage interest rates are variable. Even though the borrower is not making loan payments, upward trends in interest rates over time can slow the buildup of equity in the property. This would lessen the amount of money ultimately available to the borrower.

I would recommend using part of the proceeds from a reverse mortgage to purchase long term care insurance. This would help counter some of the risks by securing coverage of long term care expenses that would otherwise require a direct spend down of assets.

We recently had a family interested in moving their mother into one of our assisted living properties. During the tour, we learned that the original plan was to sell mom's home and use the proceeds to fund her care. However, while gathering the necessary documents to initiate the process, they discovered that mom had taken out a reverse mortgage several years earlier. Due to a significant decline in home values in her area, she had very little equity in her home. Had they discussed this with her much earlier and been familiar with her financial situation, they could have assisted her in effectively planning her future.

Reverse mortgages can also be used to provide monthly income, however, be mindful that the credit will, at some point, be exhausted. The best use of at least a portion of reverse mortgage proceeds is to purchase long term care insurance, an annuity, or to pay off existing debt.

While the traditional reverse mortgage offers seniors several ways to access equity, the requirement to remain in the home is not always the best option. The quality of the neighborhood may have deteriorated, or perhaps upkeep is simply too much of a burden. On a positive note, there are circumstances under which a home equity conversion mortgage can be used to purchase a new primary residence. This requires that the borrower/buyer is able to use cash-on-hand to pay the difference between the loan proceeds and the sales price, plus closing costs for the new residence.

One residential option is patio homes for independent living in an age-qualified, gated community. This concept is for seniors who still want to own their own home, but prefer to downsize. They can also simplify their expenses by bundling the cost of utilities and upkeep in to a single, affordable monthly regime fee.

Just last year, we facilitated a transaction where a senior adult was able to purchase one of our patio homes with a new home equity conversion mortgage product, called a reverse mortgage for purchase. This twist on the home equity conversion mortgage does not require that the borrower own the property outright, provided they can pay down enough to enable the reverse mortgage proceeds to pay the purchase price balance in full.

For almost a year, we had been working with a lady to determine how we could assist her in moving into our community. She had, for some time, wrestled with some of the typical challenges facing many senior homeowners. She constantly struggled to maintain the home, pay her monthly mortgage, utilities and other basic living costs. Social security, which was her sole source of income, fell short of covering her basic needs.

Although she had lived in the home for many years, her mortgage was unusually high, around $97,000, due to some improvements and repairs made in recent years. Her home's condition caused it to be valued at only about $170,000. The patio home was priced around $130,000.

Her challenge was twofold. Because her income was so low, she could not continue to bear a monthly mortgage payment. And because she didn't have enough equity built up, she couldn't have afforded to buy the patio home by simply selling her house.

But the reverse mortgage for purchase ended up being the perfect solution for her. By selling her home, she was able to apply $50,000 of her net proceeds as a down payment for the patio home. This was enough to qualify her for the new loan product, and the reverse mortgage paid the balance. As a result, she was able to move into her new home with no monthly mortgage payment. So now her monthly income is sufficient to cover her living expenses. Being able to escape the financial and emotional burden of her former home was a huge relief for her. She now spends her time enjoying her new home and neighbors in the Agapé Village.

Chapter 22:
Veterans Administration Benefits

The first step in pursuing Veterans Administration (VA) benefits is to determine eligibility. Spouses of veterans are eligible for some benefits. Most VA benefits are based on financial criteria, but healthcare, including assisted living and skilled nursing, are excluded from the income criteria. If you think that there is any chance that your parent may qualify for VA benefits, I encourage you to look into the matter further. Knowledge is powerful. A recent study commissioned by the VA suggested that only one-fourth of eligible veterans and about 17 percent of eligible widows are participating. [24]

A couple of years ago, we were contacted by a gentleman who had heard me speak on the radio about VA benefits. After hearing the interview, he called the county veterans affairs office and learned that his mother was eligible for $1,000 monthly assisted living benefit. He previously had delayed moving her because they had not been able to figure out how to cover the related expenses. The VA benefit, combined with her social security and retirement checks made the move to assisted living financially possible and got his mom the assistance she needed.

The VA's Aid and Attendance Program:

- Any war-time veteran with 90 days of active duty is eligible to apply for the Aid & Attendance Improved Pension. The surviving spouse of a war-time veteran may also apply. The applicant must qualify both medically and financially.

- The Aid and Attendance Improved Pension can provide up to $1,632 per month to a veteran, $1,055 per month to a surviving spouse, or $1,949 per month to a couple.

- Applicants must complete the Veterans Application for Pension or Compensation. The completed application must include a copy of the separation papers, a medical evaluation from an attending physician, a list of current medical issues, and current financial information.

- The Aid and Attendance Improved Pension provides benefits for veterans and surviving spouses who require regular assistance in eating, bathing, dressing and/or toileting. It also covers individuals who are blind or who suffer from mental or physical incapacity. Care in an assisting living facility can be covered by the Aid and Attendance Improved Pension.

- It typically takes four to six months for an application to be processed. Depending on caseload, the time frame can be much longer.

  ———————————————————————

Chapter 23:
Annuities

Annuities can be a very effective way to ensure guaranteed lifetime income for your parent. A convenient time to purchase an annuity is after selling a home or cashing out through a reverse mortgage. Some annuities also have a cash payout value upon the death of the final holder. Our insurance agency recently sold an annuity that pays a senior $600 per month for the rest of her life. The policy also extends the $600 per month lifetime income benefit to her daughter as the beneficiary. In addition, it will provide a cash benefit at the time of the daughter's death.

Chapter 24:
Transfer of Assets

For those who are fortunate enough to have accumulated significant financial and other assets, many will consider transferring these assets to their children. While some financial planners may offer advice regarding these matters, I would suggest persons transfer assets only under the advisement of an accountant or attorney who specializes in estate planning. If this type of professional is not affordable, then it is likely the individual does not have enough assets to warrant transferring assets for the purpose of avoiding inheritance taxes. Keep in mind, however, that transferring assets for the purpose of qualifying for Medicaid is considered fraudulent, and, if discovered, will result in the denial of qualification and benefits until the assets in question would have been exhausted. In any case, it is imperative that your parent understand the possible ramifications of transferring assets.

I knew a church member whose son convinced her to transfer her land into his name so that in the event she became ill she would qualify for Medicaid. Unfortunately the son's business turned sour; he lost his business and her land and her home. After having acquired a considerable amount of assets during her life, she spent her last 15 years in a very small mobile home.

Conclusion

My Closing Thoughts

The probable reality is that you have read this book because you are, or soon will be, facing the daunting task of finding suitable care for an elderly parent. You are likely anxious, confused, and even frightened at the thought of being responsible for a loved one who once took care of you. But hopefully, because of your relationship with this person, you recognize that above all else you are charged with helping them retain dignity and value throughout the remainder of their life. I trust that this book has provided you information to assist in addressing your loved one's needs; I hope that its pages have inspired you to learn even more about effective care options for senior adults; and I pray that its message will guide you in fulfilling God's challenges for you as *your loved one's keeper.*

Reference

Citations, Glossary and Helpful Contact Information

1 Belden, Nancy, John Russonello, and Kate Stewart. "In the Middle: A Report on Multicultural Boomers Coping With Family and Aging Issues." *AARP*. AARP, July 2001. Web. 8 Dec 2010. <http://assets.aarp.org/rgcenter/il/in_the_middle.pdf>.

2 Leinhard, John H. "IGNAZ PHILIPP SEMMELWEIS." *Semmelweis University English Language Program.* DataWeb Systems, 2010. Web. 8 Dec 2010. <http://www.semmelweis-english-program.org/index.php?option=com_content&task=view&id=80&Itemid=64>.

3 "Traffic Saftey Facts 2006 Data: Occupant Protection." *National Highway Traffic Safety Administration.* NHTSA, Apr 2007. Web. 8 Dec 2010. <http://www-nrd.nhtsa.dot.gov/Pubs/810807.PDF>.

4 Kusserow, Richard P. "Medication Regimens: Causes of Noncompliance." *U.S. Department of Health & Human Services: Office of Inspector General.* HHSOIG, June 1990. Web. 8 Dec 2010. <http://oig.hhs.gov/oei/reports/oei-04-89-89121.pdf>.

5 Greeley, Alexander. "Nutrition and the elderly - includes related article on recipes for a long, healthy life." *BNET.* CBS Interactive, Oct 1990.

Web. 8 Dec 2010. <http://findarticles.com/p/ articles/mi_m1370/is_n8_v24/ai_9073342/>.

6 Spurlock, Morgan, Dir. Super Size Me. Dir. Morgan Spurlock." Perf. Spurlock, Morgan. Samuel Goldwyn Films: 2004, Film. <http://super-size-me.morganspurlock.com/>.

7 Domrose, Cathryn. "Nurse-Led Efforts Aim to Reduce Hospital Readmissions." *Nurse. com.* Gannett Healthcare Group, Apr 2010. Web. 8 Dec 2010. <http://news.nurse.com/ article/20100419/NATIONAL01/104190035>.

8 Brink, Susan. "Hospice, palliative care aim to ease suffering." *MSNBC.* MSNBC, 26 Feb 2010. Web. 8 Dec 2010. <http://www.msnbc.msn. com/id/35610331>.

9 "Statistics about Accidental injury ." *CureResearch.* Health Grades, Inc., n.d. Web. 8 Dec 2010. <http://www.cureresearch.com/a/accidents/ stats.htm>.

10 Wilson, James R.M., Michael G. Clarke, Paul Ewings, John D. Graham, and Ruaraidh MacDonagh. "The assessment of patient life-expectancy: how accurate are urologists and oncologists?." *BJU International* 95.6 (2005): 794-98. Web. 8

Dec 2010. <http://onlinelibrary.wiley.com/doi/10.1111/j.1464-410X.2005.05403.x/full>.

11 The Writing Group for the SUPPORT Investigators. "A Controlled Trial to Improve Care." *Journal of the American Medical Association* 274.20 (1995): 1591-98. Web. 9 Dec 2010. <http://jama.ama-assn.org/content/274/20/1591.full.pdf+html>.

12 Marchione, Marilynn. "Many Americans over-treated to death." *MSNBC*. MSNBC, 06 Jul 2010. Web. 8 Dec 2010. <http://www.msnbc.msn.com/id/37907548/ns/health-cancer/>.

13 Marco, Catherine A., Nancy Buderer, and Dorothy Thum Sr. "End-of-life care: Perspectives of family members of deceased patients." *American Journal of Hospice and Palliative Medicine* 22.1 (2005): 26-31. Web. 8 Dec 2010. <http://ajh.sagepub.com/content/22/1/26.abstract>.

14 "Exercise Associated with Reduced Risk of Dementia in Older Adults." *Alzheimer's Disease Education and Referral Center* . National Institute of Aging, 05 Feb 2009. Web. 8 Dec 2010. <http://www.nia.nih.gov/Alzheimers/ResearchInformation/NewsReleases/Archives/PR2006/PR20060116Exercise.htm>.

15 *World's Alzheimer's cases to quadruple by 2050* . Web. 9 Dec 2010. <http://www.msnbc.msn.com/id/19168359/>.

16 "MassHealth Managed Care." *The Commonwealth of Massachusetts.* The Commonwealth of Massachusetts, Nov 2008. Web. 9 Dec 2010. <http://www.mass.gov/Eeohhs2/docs/masshealth/research/hedis_2008.txt>.

17-18 Burns, A., Banerjee, S., Morris, J., Woodward, Y., Baldwin, R., Proctor, R., Tarrier, N., Pendleton, N., Sutherland, D., Andrew, G. and Horan, M. "Treatment and Prevention of Depression After Surgery for Hip Fracture in Older People: Randomized, Controlled Trials." *Journal of the American Geriatrics Society* 55.1 (2007): 75-80. Web. 9 Dec 2010. <http://onlinelibrary.wiley.com/doi/10.1111/j.1532-5415.2007.01016.x/abstract>.

19 "Exercise Associated with Reduced Risk of Dementia in Older Adults." *National Institute on Aging.* National Institute on Aging, 2006. Web. 9 Dec 2010. <http://www.nia.nih.gov/NewsAndEvents/PressReleases/PR20060116dementia.htm>.

20 "Alzheimer's Disease Facts and Figures 2007."
    Alzheimer's Association. Alzheimer's Association,
    2007. Web. 9 Dec 2010. <http://www.alz.org/na-
    tional/documents/Report_2007FactsAndFigures.
    pdf>.

21 Williams, Mark E. "UTI and Behavioral Changes
    in the Elderly." *Medscape Today.* WebMD LLC,
    15 Jul 2003. Web. 9 Dec 2010. <http://www.
    medscape.com/viewarticle/458105>.

22 Ameriks, John, and Liqian Ren. "Generating
    Guaranteed Income:." *Vanguard.* The Vanguard
    Group, Inc., 2008. Web. 9 Dec 2010. <https://
    personal.vanguard.com/pdf/icruia.pdf>.

23 Kemper, Peter, and Christopher M. Murtaugh.
    "Lifetime Use of Nursing Home Care." *New
    England Journal of Medicine* 324.9 (1991): 595-600.
    Web. 9 Dec 2010. <http://www.nejm.org/doi/
    pdf/10.1056/NEJM199102283240905>.

24 Lade, Diane C. "Little-known VA program can
    help vets with out-of-pocket." *VeteranAid.org.*
    VeteranAid.org, 16 Feb 2006. Web. 9 Dec 2010.
    <http://www.veteranaid.org/docs/AA.pdf>.

Glossary

Activities of Daily Living (ADL): Physical activities that an independent person performs during the course of a typical day: including bathing, dressing, eating, toileting, and transferring into and out of bed.

Acute: A sudden and severe condition (e.g. a stroke or heart attack)

Administrator: A licensed professional who oversees the operation of a care facility such as a nursing home or assisted living facility.

Advance Directives: A written statement detailing an individual's preferences and directions regarding health and end-of-life care.

Age-Associated Memory Impairment: Mild memory loss that increases with age and is a normal part of the aging process.

Alzheimer's Disease: A progressive disease, typically occurring in the elderly and leading to the degeneration of the brain cells. Symptoms include severe memory loss, disorientation and inability to concentrate.

Ambulate: To walk or move about.

Aphasia: The loss of ability to communicate.

Apraxia: The inability to perform activities that an individual is physically able of accomplishing.

Assessment: Determination of a resident's care needs, based on a professional evaluation of the resident's physical and psychological condition.

Assisted Living: Senior housing that provides apartments for individuals or couples as well as assistance with activities of daily living. Facilities offer on-site staff, congregate dining, and activity programs.

Attending Physician: The physician identified by the patient as having primary responsibility for the patient's medical care.

Bed Sores: A painful, reddened area of skin resulting from pressure and lack of movement.

Bedfast: To be bed-ridden.

Benefit Period: The period of time specified in the Schedule of Benefits during which covered services are rendered and benefit maximums, deductibles and coinsurance limits are accumulated. The first and/or last benefit periods may be less than 12 months depending on the effective date and the date your coverage terminates.

Bereavement Services: The supportive services provided to family members to assist in coping with the patient's death, including follow-up assessment and assistance through the first year after death.

Board and Care Homes: These are group living arrangements that are designed to meet the needs of people who cannot live independently, but do not require nursing facility services. These facilities offer a wider range of services than independent living options. Most provide help with some of the activities of daily living. In some cases, private long term care insurance and medical-assistance programs will help pay for this type of living.

Caregiver: Any individual who takes care of an elderly person or someone with physical or mental limitations.

Cerebrovascular Accident (CVA): An event in which an area of the brain is damaged due to a sudden interruption of blood supply.

Certificate of Medical Necessity: A document completed and signed by a physician to certify a patient's need for durable medical equipment (e.g. wheelchairs, walkers, etc.) or services (e.g. assisted living, skilled nursing).

Certified Home Health Care: An entity that provides, as a minimum, the following services that are of a preventative, therapeutic, health guidance and/ or supportive nature to persons at home: nursing services; home health aide services; medical supplies, equipment and appliances suitable for use in the home; and at least one additional service such as, the provision of physical therapy, occupational therapy, speech/language pathology, respiratory therapy, nutritional services and social work services.

Certified Nursing Assistant (CNA): A CNA provides personal assistance to residents or patients, including bathing, dressing, transporting and other essential activities. CNAs are certified and work under the supervision of an RN or LPN.

Chronic: A prolonged illness or disease.

Chronic Obstructive Pulmonary Disease (COPD): A group of chronic respiratory disorders characterized by the restricted flow of air to and from the lungs.

Cognitive Impairment: A diminished mental capacity.

Cognitive Skills: Mental abilities that facilitate interaction and response.

Co-morbidities: Multiple medical conditions or disease processes.

Congestive Heart Failure (CHF): A common type of heart disease in which the heart is incapable of pumping necessary amounts of blood to body tissues.

Conservator: A court-appointed representative for a person who is mentally or physically incapable of managing his or her own legal affairs.

Continuing Care Retirement Communities (CCRCs): Housing communities that provide different levels of care based on the needs of their residents — from independent living apartments to skilled nursing in an affiliated nursing facility. Residents may move from one setting to another as their needs change, but remain in the CCRC's community.

Continuous Care: Hospice level of care in which a hospice client experiences an acute medical or psychosocial crisis requiring the presence of a hospice nurse or aide for a minimum of eight hours up to twenty hours per day for relief of acute symptoms.

Custodial Care: Personal assistance services that may or may not include a skilled nursing care component. When and if a patient is designated to custodial care, Medicare payments typically cease.

Dementia: Progressive mental disorder that affects memory, judgment and cognitive powers. One type of dementia is Alzheimer's disease.

Diagnostic Related Groups (DRGs): DRGs are used to determine the amount that Medicare reimburses hospitals for in-patient services.

Director of Nursing (DON): Oversees all nursing staff and is responsible for maintaining nursing policies and monitoring the quality of care delivered. The DON also assures compliance with state and federal guidelines.

Discharge Planner: A social worker or nurse who assists patients and their families with healthcare arrangements following a hospital stay. The discharge planner plays a pivotal role in making sure that patients are discharged to appropriate levels of care.

Do Not Resuscitate (DNR) Order: An order entered by the attending physician that states that in the event the resident suffers cardiac or respiratory arrest, cardio-pulmonary resuscitation (CPR) should not be attempted.

Dual Eligibility: Qualification for both Medicaid and Medicare.

Durable Power of Attorney for Healthcare (DPAHC): A legal document in which a competent person gives another person the power to make healthcare decisions, should the former become unable to make those decisions.

Dysphagia: A swallowing disorder that hinders the movement of food from the mouth to the stomach.

Edema: A collection of fluid in the tissues which causes swelling.

Eden Alternative: A concept for skilled nursing facilities that embraces children, nature and animals to be part of facility life.

Emergency Response Systems: Electronic monitors on a person or in a home that automatically signal for medical response teams in cases of duress.

End Stage Renal Disease (ESRD): A medical condition in which a person's kidneys shut down, requiring the individual to receive dialysis or a kidney transplant.

Fee for Service: A method of charging whereby a medical practitioner bills for each service rendered.

Fee Schedule: A listing of agreed-upon charges or established allowances for specified medical procedures.

Geriatrics: The branch of medicine that focuses on providing health-care for the elderly.

Grandfather: A legal term signifying that all existing conditions that were present at the time of a law or legal agreement can be exempted since they were in place when the conditions were legal.

Guardianship: A measure that severely restricts (and transfers) the legal rights of an elder based on a court's finding of legal incompetence.

Healthcare Directive: A written legal document which allows a person to appoint another person to make healthcare or end-of-life decisions should the former become incapable of making decisions.

Healthcare Power of Attorney: The appointment of a health-care agent to make decisions when an individual becomes unable to make decisions.

Health Maintenance Organization (HMO): An organization that provides a range of healthcare services to its subscribers.

Home Health Agency (HHA): An agency that provides medical services in a home setting. Services may be provided by a nurse, a therapist, a social worker, or any combination of these service providers.

Home Health Aide: An aide who provides personal care such as bathing, dressing and grooming for home-bound individuals.

Hospice: A public agency or private organization providing terminally ill patients a centrally-administered plan of care that emphasizes comfort through symptom management.

Incident: Any event or occurrence having the potential for causing harm to an individual.

Incompetence: A legal term used to describe an individual who is, due to mental deficiencies, incapable of managing his or her own affairs.

Incontinent: Unable to control bladder and/or bowel functions.

Inpatient: A patient who has been admitted, on an overnight basis, to a hospital or other health facility for the purpose of receiving a diagnosis, treatment, or other health services.

Interdisciplinary Team: A group designated by a facility to provide or supervise care, treatment, and services provided by the facility. The team typically includes two or more of the following professionals: a registered nurse, dietician, social worker and nursing aide.

Intermediate Care Facility/Mentally Retarded (ICF/MR): A licensed facility providing health or rehabilitative services for people with stable, chronic developmental disabilities.

Living Will: A legal document in which a person provides explicit instructions regarding which medical treatments should (and should not) be used in case of a terminal injury or illness.

Long Term Care (LTC): The broad spectrum of medical and support services available to persons whose independence has been compromised due to chronic illness or condition. Long term care can consist of in-home care, adult day healthcare, or care in assisted living or skilled nursing facilities.

Long Term Care Insurance: Insurance designed to assist with the costs associated with long term care.

Managed Care: A method of financing and providing healthcare for a set fee using a network of medical professionals.

Medicaid: The federal public assistance program that pays for healthcare services for low income, elderly, or disabled persons who qualify.

Medicaid-Certified Bed: A bed in a nursing facility that meets federal standards for Medicaid recipients.

Medical Director: The individual who oversees medical-care operations for an office or facility.

Medicare: The federal program that provides primarily skilled medical care for people aged 65 and older.

Medicare Part A: Government administered insurance that helps pay for inpatient hospital care, short-term rehabilitation, hospice care, and some home health care for seniors.

Medicare Part B: Government administered insurance that helps pay for doctors' services and outpatient hospital care.

Medicare Part C: Insurance that combines Parts "A" and "B" services and is provided through commercial insurance companies. (Benefits vary by plan.)

Medicare Part D: Government administered prescription drug coverage.

Medicare Supplemental Insurance: Private insurance (often called "Medigap") that covers Medicare's deductibles and co-insurances.

Medicare-Certified Bed: A nursing facility bed in a building that meets federal standards for Medicare patients who require skilled nursing care.

Nurse, Licensed Practical (LPN): A graduate of a practical nursing education program who has passed a state examination and is licensed to provide nursing and personal care under the supervision of a registered nurse or physician.

Nurse, Registered (RN): A graduate from a formal program of nursing education who has passed a state-administered exam. RNs have completed more formal training than licensed practical nurses and have a wide scope of responsibility including all aspects of nursing care.

Nursing Facility (NF): A facility providing nursing services and rehabilitative care, including physical, occupational or speech therapy. (See Skilled Nursing Facility, Nursing Home.)

Nursing Home: A facility providing nursing services and rehabilitative care, including physical, occupational or speech therapy. (See Skilled Nursing Facility.)

Occupational Therapist: A therapist who evaluates, treats, and consults with individuals whose abilities to manage the tasks of daily life have been reduced by physical illness or injury, psychosocial disability, or developmental deficits.

Ombudsman Program: A program that protects the rights of all residents in 24-hour long term care facilities. A key component of the Ombudsman Program is a collective of volunteers who monitor local facilities, observe conditions of care and attempt to resolve issues of conflict with staff.

Outpatient: A patient who receives care at a healthcare facility without being admitted to the facility.

Palliative Care: A system of symptom management that incorporates medical, nursing, psychosocial, and spiritual care according to the needs, values, beliefs, and culture or cultures of the patient and his or her family. Palliative care is intended to achieve relief from, reduction of, or elimination of pain and of other physical, emotional, social, or spiritual symptoms of distress.

Personal Care: Services provided by a nurse's aide, dietician or other health professional. Assistance with walking, getting out of bed, bathing, toileting, dressing and eating may be part of personal care.

Physical Therapy: Services provided by therapists in order to relieve pain, restore maximum strength and flexibility, and prevent additional injury.

Power of Attorney: A legal document allowing one person to act in a legal matter on another's behalf regarding legal matters.

Pre-Admission Screening: An assessment of an individual's needs in order to determine what type of facility (if any) the individual should be placed.

Pressure Ulcers: See bed sores.

Primary Care: Care provided by physicians specifically trained for and skilled in comprehensive first contact and continuing care for persons with any undiagnosed sign, symptom, or health concern not limited by problem origin (biological, behavioral, or social), organ system, or diagnosis.

Private Pay Patients: Patients who pay for their own care or whose care is paid for by an insurance company. The term is used to distinguish patients from those whose care is paid for by government programs such as Medicaid or Medicare.

Provider: Someone who provides medical services or supplies.

Representative: An individual who has been authorized under state law to terminate an individual's medical care or to elect or revoke the election of hospice care on behalf of a terminally ill individual who is mentally or physically incapacitated.

Resident Care Plan: A written plan of care for residents or patients, which specifies measurable objectives and timetables for services to be provided to meet a resident's needs. (Also referred to as "care plan".)

Respiratory Therapy: Therapy for patients with breathing difficulties.

Respite Care: Care provided on a temporary basis to an individual who needs nursing facility care, but who is normally cared for at home. The goals of respite care are to provide care for the patient as well as to provide rest for the patient's caregiver(s).

Routine Home Care: A routine home care day on which a hospice client who has elected to receive hospice care is at home and is not receiving continuous care, respite care or general inpatient care.

Skilled Nursing Facility (SNF): A facility that provides nursing services and rehabilitative care, including physical, occupational or speech therapy.

Speech Therapy: Therapy designed to help individuals overcome conditions such as speaking and swallowing difficulties.

Terminally Ill: A state in which therapeutic intervention directed toward cure of the disease is no longer appropriate and the patient's medical prognosis is one in which there is a life expectancy of six months or less.

Helpful Contact Information

Please note that some of the following information pertains solely to South Carolina organizations, however, each state likely has similar entities. Non-SC residents should research the availability of such services within their respective state.

Agencies, Bureau's and Commissions

Alzheimer's Resource Coordination Center
www.aging.sc.gov/seniors/alzheimersresourceco-ordinationcenter/
(803) 734-9900

Center for Disease Control
www.cdc.gov
(800) 232-4636

Center for Food Safety
www.centerforfoodsafety.org
(202) 547-9359

Department of Health and Human Services
www.hhs.gov
(877) 696-6775

Developmental Disabilities Association
www.develop.bc.ca
(604) 273-9778

Food & Drug Administration
www.fda.gov
(888) 463-6332

Healthcare Compliance Association
www.hcca-info.org
(888) 580-8373

Health Professionals Bureau
bhpr.hrsa.gov
(952) 988-0141

National AIDS Clearinghouse
www.unesco.org/en/aids

National Cancer Institute
www.cancer.gov
(800) 422-6237

National Center for Health Statistics
fedstats.gov

National Health Information Center
health.gov/nhic

National Institute of Mental Health
nimh.nih.gov
(866) 615-6464

National Institute on Aging
www.nia.nih.gov
(800) 222-2225

National Institute of Health
nih.gov
(301) 496-4000

National Library of Medicine
www.nlm.nih.gov
(888) 346-3656

OSHA
osha.gov
(800) 321-6742

Social Security Administration
ssa.gov
(800) 772-1213

Healthcare Organizations

American Medical Association
www.ama-assn.org
(800) 621-8335

American Women's Medical Association
www.amwa-doc.org
(215) 320-3716

South Carolina Associations and Organizations

SC Area Health Education Consortium
scahec.net
(843) 792-4431

SC Health Alliance
scha.org
(843) 681-6122

SC Healthcare Association
schca.org
(843) 681-6122

SC Healthcare Human Resources Association
scha.org
(803) 796-3080

South Carolina Government Agencies

Department of Health and Environmental Control
www.scdhec.gov
(803) 898-3432

Insurance Counseling Assistance
& Referrals for Elders
aging.sc.gov/seniors/icare.htm
(803) 898-2850

National Council on Aging
ncoa.org
(202) 479-1200

Office of Veterans Affairs
www.govoepp.state.sc.us/va
(800) 827-1000

Ombudsman's Program
aging.sc.gov/seniors/ombudsman.htm
(803) 734-9900

SC Department of DSS
www.state.sc.us/dss
(803) 898-7601

SC Department of Health and Human Services
www.dhhs.state.sc.us
(888) 549-0820

SC Department of Labor, Licensing and Regulations
llr.state.sc.us
(803) 896-4300

SC Department of Mental Health
www.state.sc.us/dmh
(803) 898-8581

SC Human Affairs Commission
www.state.sc.us/schac
(803) 737-7800

Hospice

American Association of Home Care
nahc.org
(202) 547-7424

American Society on Aging
asaging.org
(415) 974-0300

Hospice Foundation of America
hospicefoundation.org
(800) 854-3402

National Hospice and Palliative Care Association
nhpco.org
(703) 837-1500

National Association of Home Care and Hospice
nahc.org
(202) 547-7424

Long Term Care Resources

*American Association of Homes
and Service for the Aging*
aahsa.org
(202) 783-2242

American Healthcare Association
www.ahca.org
(202) 842-4444

ElderWeb
elderweb.com
(780) 468-1985

Long Term Care Link
longtermcarelink.net
(801) 298-8676

Bereavement, Grief, Death and Dying

Association for Death Education and Counseling
www.adec.org
(847) 509-0403

Caring Connections
caringinfo.org
(800) 658-8898

HospiceNet
hospicenet.org
(615) 371-9363

National Associations and Organizations

Assisted Living Federation of America
www.alfa.org
(703) 894-1805

Meals on Wheels Association of America
www.mowaa.org
(730) 548-8024

National Association of Elder Law Attorneys
www.naela.org
(703) 942-5711

*National Association of Professional
Geriatric Care Managers*
caremanager.org
(520) 881-8008

National Association of Senior Move Managers
nasmm.org
(877) 606-2766

National Center on Elder Abuse
ncea.aoa.gov
(800) 677-1116

National Family Care Givers Association
thefamilycaregiver.org
(800) 896-3650

Health, Medical and Pharmaceutical Resources

Alzheimer's Association
alz.org
(800) 272-3900

National Institute of Mental Health
nimh.nih.gov
(301) 443-4513

RxList
www.rxlist.com

Consumer Reports
www.BestBuyDrugs.org

eMedicineHealth
www.emedicinehealth.com